Lung Cancer 1982

Lung Cancer 1982

General Lectures and Special Topics presented at
The III World Conference on Lung Cancer,
Tokyo, Japan, May 17–20, 1982

Editors:

Shichiro Ishikawa
National Cancer Center, Tokyo

Yoshihiro Hayata
Tokyo Medical College, Tokyo

Keiichi Suemasu
National Cancer Center, Tokyo

 1982

Excerpta Medica, Amsterdam-Oxford-Princeton

International Congress Series No. 569
ISBN Excerpta Medica 90 219 0569 8
ISBN Elsevier North-Holland 0 444 90238 4

Library of Congress Cataloging in Publication Data

World Conference on Lung Cancer (3rd : 1982 : Tokyo,
    Japan)
    Lung cancer 1982.

    1. Lungs--Cancer--Congresses. I. Ishikawa, Shichirō,
1910-   . II. Title. [DNLM: 1. Lung neoplasma--
Congresses. W3 EX89 no.569 1982 / WF 658 W926 1982L]
RC280.L8W65 1982   616.99'424   82-2484
ISBN 90-219-0569-8   AACR2
ISBN 0-444-90238-4 (Elsevier North-Holland)

Publisher:
Excerpta Medica
305 Keizersgracht
1000 BC Amsterdam
P.O. Box 1126

Sole Distributors for the USA and Canada:
Elsevier North-Holland Inc.
52 Vanderbilt Avenue
New York, N.Y. 10017

Printed in Japan

Contributors

M. Aida
Department of Surgery,
Tokyo Medical College,
6-7-1, Nishishinjuku,
Shinjuku-ku,
Tokyo 160,
Japan

N.M. Bleehen
University Department and Medical Research
Council Unit of Clinical Oncology
and Radiotherapeutics,
The Medical School,
Cambridge CB2 2QQ,
United Kingdom

D.N. Carney
NCI-Navy Medical Oncology Branch,
National Cancer Institute
and National Naval Medical Center,
Bethesda, MD 20814,
U.S.A.

A.F. Gazdar
NCI-Navy Medical Oncology Branch,
National Cancer Institute
and National Naval Medical Center,
Bethesda, MD 20814,
U.S.A.

H.H. Hansen
Chemotherapy Department R II-V,
Finsen Institute,
Strandboulevarden 49,
DK-2100 Copenhagen,
Denmark

C.C. Harris
Laboratory of Human Carcinogenesis,
National Cancer Institute,
Bethesda, MD 21205
U.S.A.

Y. Hayata
Department of Surgery,
Tokyo Medical College,
6-7-1, Nishishinjuku,
Shinjuku-ku,
Tokyo 160,
Japan

T. Hirayama
Epidemiology Division,
National Cancer Center,
Research Institute,
Tsukiji,
Tokyo 104,
Japan

H. Kato
Department of Surgery,
Tokyo Medical College,
6-7-1, Nishishinjuku,
Shinjuku-ku,
Tokyo 160,
Japan

C. Konaka
Department of Surgery,
Tokyo Medical College,
6-7-1, Nishishinjuku,
Shinjuku-ku,
Tokyo 160,
Japan

J.D. Minna
NCI-Navy Medical Oncology Branch,
National Cancer Institute
and National Naval Medical Center,
Bethesda, MD 20814,
U.S.A.

K. Nishimiya
Department of Surgery,
Tokyo Medical College,
6-7-1, Nishishinjuku,
Shinjuku-ku,
Tokyo 160,
Japan

J. Ono
Department of Surgery,
Tokyo Medical College,
6-7-1, Nishishinjuku,
Shinjuku-ku,
Tokyo 160,
Japan

B.F. Trump
Department of Pathology,
University of Maryland,
School of Medicine,
10 S. Pine Street,
Baltimore, MD 21201,
U.S.A.

T. Wilson
Department of Pathology,
University of Maryland,
School of Medicine,
10 S. Pine Street,
Baltimore, MD 21201,
U.S.A.

Introduction

On the occasion of the III Conference on Lung Cancer, in Tokyo in 1982, being held under the auspices of the International Association for the Study of Lung Cancer (IASLC), three General Lectures and three Special Topics have been arranged. These Lectures and Topics are not only of current interest but are also of practical importance in the field of lung cancer research. Those who are giving these talks are distinguished scientists at the forefront of their respective fields. Their generous contribution to this Conference is greatly appreciated.

Although through steady efforts the results of lung cancer treatment are improving gradually, the average cure rate in Japan still remains at only 14%, according to the data reported in 1980. It will therefore be necessary to expend even more strenuous efforts to achieve early detection by improving diagnostic methods, and by the use of X-rays and endoscopy as well as laser and tumor markers. It goes without saying that mass-screening must be carried out effectively. On the other hand, in daily practice we are faced with a large number of patients with advanced lung cancer. For these patients, it is very important that new chemotherapeutic agents be developed, that the best combinations of these agents be determined, and that various methods such as immune therapy, irradiation, thermotherapy and laser therapy be used.

At the same time, it is a matter of urgency that the actual causes of lung cancer be identified and that ways to prevent its occurrence be established. For this purpose, basic research as well as a detailed epidemiological survey for each patient (bedside epidemiology) will become increasingly important in the future.

The purpose of this booklet is to provide comprehensive and up-to-date information for those actually engaged in the research, diagnosis and treatment of lung cancer and for all who are otherwise interested in these areas.

Finally, I sincerely hope that this Conference, which is being attended by experts from all over the world, will prove to be a milestone in the conquest of lung cancer.

Shichiro Ishikawa
Tokyo, March 1982

Contents

Epidemiological aspects of lung cancer in the Orient

Takeshi Hirayama

The available information on the epidemiology of lung cancer in the Orient will be summarized under the following headings: (1) patterns of occurrence, (2) host factors, (3) environmental factors and (4) strategies for control.

Patterns of occurrence

Time trends

The mortality due to lung cancer has been increasing rapidly. Until a few years ago, the number of deaths in Japan from pulmonary tuberculosis was far higher than that from lung cancer. As registered in 1947, the death toll due to pulmonary tuberculosis was 121,912, which was 152 times that registered for lung cancer (768 cases). This balance has decreased each year. In 1972, the number of pulmonary tuberculosis deaths (11,983) was lower than the number of lung cancer deaths (12,290). The figures were 6144 and 21,294, respectively, in 1980. If the current pace continues, the death rate for lung cancer is expected to catch up, within a decade at the latest, with that of stomach cancer in Japan. The death rates are on the increase in each age group in both males and females. It is noteworthy that the rate has been increasing even in cohorts born in 1940–1944, which suggests that a limited effect of low-tar cigarettes has appeared since 1965, the cumulative mortality rate for lung cancer by age 39 being 3.2, 3.6 and 4.5 per 100,000 in cohorts born in 1930–1934, 1935–1939 and 1940–1944, respectively (1). This increasing incidence and mortality are seen in nearly all countries, including those of the Orient.

In Shanghai, the standardized mortality rates for lung cancer in males were 28.5, 44.2 and 52.0 per 100,000 in 1963–1965, 1972–1975 and 1976–1979, respectively. In females, the rates were 11.1, 16.8 and 18.3, respectively (Gao Yu-Tong).

In Singapore Chinese, the standardized lung-cancer incidence rates were 12.9, 56.9 and 68.0 per 100,000 in 1950–1961, 1968–1972 and 1973–1977, respectively. In females, the rates were 3.2, 17.3 and 20.0, respectively (Cancer Registry, Singapore).

In Korea, the relative frequencies of lung cancer to cancer of all sites were 4.1%, 11.2% and 12.5% in 1958–1967 (Ref. 11), in 1975 (Ref. 12) and in 1979 (Ref. 13), respectively, in 10,408, 2382 and 1279 males. In females, the percentages were 0.7, 2.7 and 3.6, respectively, in 16,513, 2584 and 1263 cases.

In the Philippines, the relative frequencies of lung cancer were 6.9%, 13.5% and 19.9% in 1958–1967, 1968–1973 and 1977, respectively, in 771, 6771 and 1258 males. In females, the percentages were 1.2, 3.0 and 6.1 in 1309, 9721 and 1409 cases, respectively (Philippine Cancer Society).

In the Radiotherapy Department, Postgraduate Institute, Chandigarh, India, the relative frequencies of lung cancer were 6.1%, 7.7%, 8.0% and 10.0% in 1971, 1974, 1977 and 1980, respectively, in males out of 525, 752, 789 and 813 male cancer cases. The percentages for females were 1.4, 0.3, 0.1 and 0.8, respectively, in 592, 556, 808 and 987 cancer cases.

In most developed countries, mortality among females is increasing rapidly, while in males it is less steep or almost saturating, thus reflecting different trends in smoking habits. In the Orient, however, the disease is generally on the increase, in both males and females, thus reflecting similar trends in smoking habits.

International variations

The highest rates of lung cancer are found in the United Kingdom and Finland, the lowest in Asia and Africa (2, 3). The variation is generally less in females. Roughly speaking, these rates parallel both the diagnostic level and prevalence of cigarette-smoking in each country.

Clustering within countries

Clustering is almost universally noted in urban areas, again probably reflecting the higher prevalence of smoking plus the combined effect of high-risk occupations and possibly also of indoor and outdoor air pollution. The lung cancer map recently made in China is also in line with the tendency in other countries.

Migration

Rates for immigrants from low-risk areas tend gradually to converge to the risk of the host country. This tendency is particularly marked when people from low-risk areas migrate to cities or countries with a high prevalence of cigarette-smoking (4).

Host factors

Sex

Relatively speaking, a lower sex ratio in lung cancer is a feature in Asia. However, in Europe and North America, the ratio is falling, with a more rapid increase in incidence in females.

Age

A steep rise is seen with increasing age. A linear increase is observed on a log-log graph.

Genetic predisposition

Although environmental influences predominate, there is an interaction between familial susceptibility and cigarette-smoking. Investigation of genetic differences in the inducibility of aryl hydrocarbon hydroxylase will hopefully explain some of the mechanisms of this interaction.

Precancerous lesions

Epithelial metaplasia, dysplasia and scars in lung parenchyma are regarded as precancerous lesions which would affect the cell type of carcinoma. Environmental influences, such as cigarette-smoking, must be the main factor.

Predisposing morbid conditions

A higher incidence in former tuberculosis patients is reported (15). An increased incidence of adenocarcinoma is reported (16) in patients with scleroderma, the main features being a female preponderance and a positive correlation with the intensity of sclerodermic interstitial pulmonary fibrosis.

Multiple primary neoplasms

Lung cancer appears occasionally in combination with other smoking-associated cancers (e.g. laryngeal or bladder cancer). This information is important for the prevention of secondary cancer.

Environmental factors

Socioeconomic status

A characteristic socioeconomic variation in lung cancer incidence which differs greatly in each country is probably related to the patterns of cigarette-smoking in each community. In India and Sri Lanka, people of lower socioeconomic status smoke Bidis rather than cigarettes.

Tobbaco

The association with cigarette-smoking is quite strong in males and is also significant in females. The attributable risk in males from cigarette-smoking often exceeds 70%. In females, more cases were observed to be under the influence of passive smoking. The lung cancer risk in non-smoking wives was observed to be 1.61 and 2.08 when husbands smoke 1–19 and 20 or more cigarettes daily compared to women with non-smoking husbands (prospective study, Japan) (Fig. 1) (10). Similar results were reported from Greece in a case-control study. Since side-stream smoke of cigarettes contains a higher concentration of carcinogens than main-stream smoke, these data, when further confirmed, will be of great importance for public health.

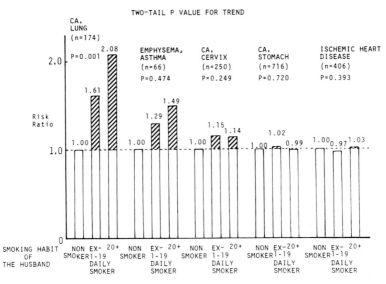

FIG. 1. *Age-occupation standardized mortality ratio for selected causes of death in non-smoking women according to smoking habits of husbands. Prospective study, Japan, 1966–1979.*

4

Tumors associated with cigarette-smoking and other air-borne carcinogens are mainly squamous-cell carcinoma and small-cell (oat-cell) carcinoma. The proportion of adenocarcinomas is higher in females. This is of interest since most passive smokers inhale side-stream smoke through the nose instead of through the mouth.

Daily cigarette-smoking proved to be the most important cause of lung cancer in Japan in the ongoing prospective study conducted by the present writer, the relative risk and attributable risk being 4.13 and 69.42%, respectively, in males. The study includes 265,118 adults aged

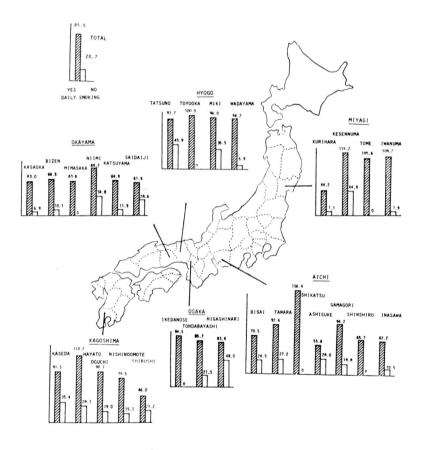

FIG. 2. *Standardized mortality rate for lung cancer according to habits of smoking and health center districts. Prospective study (males), Japan, 1966–1978.*

40 years and above comprising 91–99% of the census population in 29 health center districts. These people were interviewed from October to December, 1965 (5–7). These interviews were held at the time of the Japanese census in 1965. A record-linkage system was established between the risk-factor records (collected in 1965 and checked in 1971 and 1976), a current residence list obtained by specially planned annual census, and death certificates. During 13 years' follow-up, there have been 3,060,499 (1,369,937 males and 1,690,562 females) observed person-years. A total of 39,127 deaths occurred during this period (22,946 males and 16,181 females). The number of lung cancer deaths was 1244 (940 males and 304 females). The subjects were generally healthy at the time of interview and they were grouped according to their smoking habits into non-smokers, occasional smokers, ex-smokers and daily smokers. Standardized mortality rates of lung cancer were calculated over the 13-year period. In any of 29 health center districts where the study was performed, daily cigarette-smokers showed a far higher standardized mortality rate for lung cancer than non-smokers (Fig. 2). There was a clear-cut dose-response relationship, the standardized mortality rates for lung cancer being 20.7, 42.2, 77.0, 104.4, 141.5 and 177.6 in non-smokers, daily smokers of less than 9, 10–14, 15–24, 25–49 and

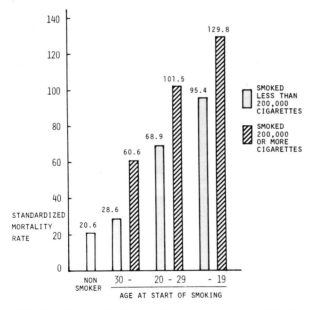

FIG. 3. *Standardized mortality rate for cancer of the lung according to age at start of smoking and total number of cigarettes smoked.*

6

50 cigarettes, respectively. For each category of cigarette-smoking, the risk was higher for those who began smoking in their teens (Fig. 3). Such early-age starters showed about 5 times higher risk of lung cancer compared to non-smokers. The fact that both the age at start of smoking and the total amount of smoking independently influence the risk of lung cancer indicates that carcinogens included in cigarette smoke must be operating both as initiators and promoters.

A similar dose-response relationship was observed in China, the Philippines and India by case-control studies.

In Buhan, China, a study conducted in 1977 on 148 males with lung cancer (diagnosed in 1974–1977) and age-matched (with 5-year range) controls (non-cancer, non-respiratory cases) revealed that the risk of cigarette-smoking was 1.00, 1.26, 1.48, 2.19 and 3.58 in non-smokers, daily smokers of less than 5, 6–10, 11–19 and 20 or more cigarettes, respectively (Buhan Medical School, 1977).

In the Philippines, case-control studies conducted by the author on 150 male lung cancer cases and 203 controls (stomach cancer) registered at the Philippine Cancer Society revealed that the relative risk was 1.00, 1.08, 1.79, 2.40, 3.43, 4.90 and 17.15 in non-smokers, daily smokers of 1–9, 10–19, 20–29, 30–39, 40–49 and 50 or more cigarettes, respectively.

In Bombay, India, case-control studies conducted on 792 pairs of lung cancer cases and matched controls showed that the relative risk was 1.0, 3.1 and 9.5, respectively, in non-smokers, daily smokers of less than 20, 20 and more cigarettes, respectively. Bidi-smoking was also reported to enhance the risk of lung cancer, the relative risk being 19.3 (Ref. 14).

Alcohol

Although there is an association with alcohol consumption, this has not been demonstrated independently of cigarette-smoking.

Diet

Vitamin A deficiency may increase the risk of lung cancer in man. Persons observed in a prospective study in Japan were divided into those who took green-yellow vegetables daily and those who did not and also by socioeconomic status. Green-yellow vegetables are defined as those containing over 1000 International Units of beta-carotine per 100 g: e.g. carrots, spinach, green pimento, pumpkin, green lettuce, chives, leek (green), turnip leaves, asparagus (green), chicory and parsley. For daily consumers of green-yellow vegetables, the age-adjusted death rates for

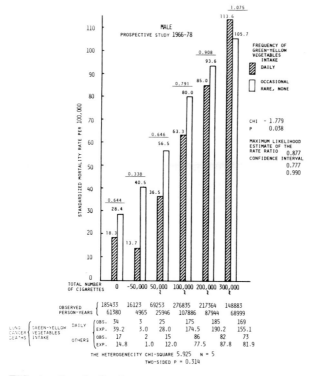

FIG. 4. *Standardized mortality rate for lung cancer according to total number of cigarettes smoked and frequency of consumption of green-yellow vegetables.*

lung cancer were 44.8 per 100,000, whereas non-daily-consumers had rates of 58.8 in higher social classes. The ratio is 0.76. This ratio increases slightly with a decrease in social status, but the risk-lowering effect remains throughout. Green-yellow vegetable consumption was then cross-tabulated with smoking: consumers of green-yellow vegetables showed a lower risk of lung cancer for both smokers and non-smokers. This was found to be significant for both males and females. There is a dose-response relationship between the total number of cigarettes ever smoked and the lung cancer risk and in each category of smoking; daily consumers of green-yellow vegetables showed a lower standardized mortality rate for lung cancer compared to non-daily consumers, except for those who had smoked over 300,000 cigarettes in the past (Fig. 4). The beneficial effect of daily consumption of green-yellow vegetables is absent in those who started smoking in their teens. From green-yellow vegetables, there is an estimated intake of 640 IU of vitamin A and 75.2 mg of vitamin C in 1970 in Japan. This amount of vitamin A is 44% of the total daily intake in Japan. The vitamin C represents 23% of the total daily intake. Thus, if green-yellow vegetables play a protective role, the main candidate must be vitamin A, followed by vitamin C, plus perhaps other unknown factors. Similar studies are expected to be conducted in other countries in the Orient.

Radiation

The lung cancer risk is reported to be high in those who work in mines with high atmospheric radon (e.g. uranium, fluorspar and hematite mines). An increased risk was also observed in patients irradiated for spondylitis. The increased risk in atomic bomb survivors in Hiroshima and Nagasaki does not seem to be explained on the basis of smoking or occupational exposure alone.

Occupation

Hazardous industries for lung cancer include uranium, hematite, fluorspar and asbestos mining, milling and manufacture of coal-gas in gas and steel works, as well as exposure to nickel and chrome ore dust.

Specific carcinogens include arsenic, asbestos, mustard gas, polycyclic aromatic hydrocarbons, radon products, and bis(chloromethyl) ether. The multiplicative effect of cigarette-smoking and asbestos exposure has been noted. Similar situations may exist with other occupational carcinogens. Each of these occupations was also found to be an important risk factor for lung cancer in Japan. For instance, metal workers were found to have a significantly higher risk of lung cancer.

Material used is derived from the Vital Statistics, 1960–1967, Japan, and the Census Report, 1965, Japan. According to the 1965 census in Japan, there were 377,100 males classified as metal workers. During the period 1960–1967, there were 39,255 lung cancer deaths. Of these, 232 lung cancer deaths occurred in metal workers. This is excessive when compared to the expected number of deaths (176.54), which was obtained by applying the age-specific mortality rates from lung cancer from each year to the age-specific census population of these workers (9). The excess deaths from lung cancer in metal workers were noted in 1960–1963 and in 1964–1967. Excess deaths from lung cancer were observed also in workers in the mining and quarrying industries (population 2,152,000). The observed number of lung cancer deaths totaled 151; expected, 127.93 ($\chi^2 = 4.16$, $P < 0.05$). No other occupations showed excess deaths from lung cancer in this study.

The higher risk of lung cancer in metal workers was also observed in the on-going prospective study in Japan. For all groups, the standardized mortality rates for lung cancer were 20.7 per 100,000 in non-smokers and 85.5 in daily cigarette-smokers. The corresponding rates for metal workers were 62.5 and 142.1, respectively. The influence was observed to be independent of the effect of cigarette-smoking.

Air pollution

Although chemicals in air-borne particles, such as nitroarenes in diesel emissions, are known to be both mutagenic and carcinogenic, the risk to humans is still controversial. There is no doubt that the lung cancer risk tends to be higher in polluted areas, but the effect has never been fully distinguished from urban-rural gradients in cigarette-smoking and the occupational risks of dust.

In our on-going prospective study in Japan, there was little difference in the standardized mortality rate for lung cancer by density of population in daily cigarette-smokers, the rates being 80.9, 89.1 and 86.9 per 100,000 in −149, 150−199 and 600− population per 1 km^2, respectively. The corresponding rates for non-smokers were 15.7, 21.5 and 26.9, showing a suggestive upward trend.

Strategies for lung cancer control

Measures against hazardous components of cigarettes

Low-tar cigarettes are now being manufactured and are progressively coming into wider use. Although the risk of lung cancer in low-tar-cigarette smokers has been shown to be significantly lower than in high-tar-cigarette smokers, the fact that lung cancer mortality is still on the increase in cohorts born after 1940−1944 who must have smoked predominantly low-tar cigarettes clearly indicates the need for caution in not being too optimistic about the control of the lung cancer epidemic by this measure alone. To reduce the risk of passive smoking, the quality control of side-stream smoke should be planned and implemented.

Measures aimed at age at first exposure

The results of studies conducted in Japan, U.S.A., U.K. and other countries have clearly shown that the age of starting cigarette-smoking is just as important as the amount of smoking in later years. The lung cancer standardized mortality rates per 100,000 were 90.6, 74.2, 35.2, 36.4 and 20.7 in those who started the habit at age 15−19, 20−24, 25−29, 30−34 and 35 or older and non-smokers, respectively, in our prospective study in Japan. Cross-tabulation by age at first starting to smoke and by the total number of cigarettes ever smoked raises the risk of lung cancer independently, suggesting that cigarette smoke plays a role as both initiator and promoter as described above. Efforts should be focussed, therefore, on making the start of exposure as late as possible.

Measures aimed at limiting exposure

Limitation of exposure and cessation could be achieved either by lowering or nullifying the size of population exposed or by lowering the amount of smoking to a minimum. In our prospective study, a clear-cut reduction in the standardized mortality rate for lung cancer was observed in ex-smokers, the risk becoming lower with the number of years after stopping smoking. The standardized mortality rates for lung cancer in males per 100,000 were 85.5, 49.9, 33.6 and 20.7, respectively, in current smokers, 1–4 years, 5 years or more after stopping smoking and in non-smokers.

Measures to reduce the risk due to passive smoking

Prohibition of smoking in public places and in closed rooms with poor ventilation should be enforced to reduce the risk of exposure to passive smoking. Another strategy is to try to remove promoters or to introduce promoter inhibitors. In our prospective study, the risk-lowering effect of the daily intake of green-yellow vegetables was clearly observed for lung cancer. The risk-lowering effect on lung cancer was observed in each category of cigarette-smoking in both sexes. This risk-lowering effect of the daily consumption of green-yellow vegetables was particularly conspicuous in ex-smokers. The standardized mortality for lung cancer observed to drop proportionally with the lapse of years after stopping smoking was far more striking in daily consumers of green-yellow vegetables than in non-daily consumers.

Early detection

Studies in the secondary prevention of lung cancer are also in progress in Japan and the U.S.A. Many early cases of lung cancer have been detected by mass-screening programs aimed at heavy smokers and other high-risk population groups (people with a family history of lung cancer). The techniques generally used are sputum cytology plus two-dimensional chest X-rays. Although the exact effect of screening on the reduction of the lung cancer death rate has not yet been demonstrated and the existing data of better survival of lung cancer cases detected by the screening are explained mainly by both lead-time bias and length bias, the program itself served as the best means of public education since it demonstrates the unbelievably higher risk of lung cancer in apparently healthy heavy-smokers.

Cost-effectiveness

The evaluation of the effect of such measures should be conducted and checked periodically using strict scientific criteria.

The validity, practicability and cost-effectiveness of each of these measures should be carefully checked, taking varying local medical and demographic conditions into consideration.

Summary

The risk of lung cancer has been increasing in recent years, particularly in those with the habit of cigarette-smoking, in most countries in the world, including the Orient. It is also high in those intensively exposed to passive smoking and to occupational carcinogens or other selected environmental agents such as arsenic, asbestos, metals and radiation. Examples of these are coming to light in certain countries in the Orient. The risk is also raised in those with a family history of this cancer.

References

1. Ministry of Health and Welfare: *Vital Statistics, 1955–1979.* Statistics and Information Department, Tokyo, Japan.
2. Waterhouse, J., Muir, C., Correa, P. and Powell, J. (Eds.) (1976): *Cancer Incidence in Five Continents, Vol. III.* Agency for Research on Cancer, Lyon.
3. Hirayama, T. (1978): Comparative epidemiology of cancer in the U.S. and Japan: morbidity. In: *The US-Japan Cooperative Cancer Research Program.* Japan Society for the Promotion of Science.
4. Wynder, E.L. and Hirayama, T. (1977): Comparative epidemiology of cancers of the United States and Japan. *Prev. Med., 6,* 567.
5. Hirayama, T. (1976): Epidemiology of lung cancer based on population studies. In: *Clinical Implications of Air Pollution Research*, pp. 69–78. American Medical Association, Chicago.
6. Hirayama, T. (1977): Smoking and cancer: a prospective study on cancer epidemiology based on census population in Japan. In: *Proceedings, III World Conference on Smoking and Health, 1975, Vol. 2*, pp. 65–72. DHEW Publ. No. 77–1413, National Institutes of Health, Bethesda, MD.
7. Hirayama, T. (1977): Prospective study on cancer epidemiology based on census population in Japan. In: *Prevention and Detection of Cancer, Part*

1: Prevention; 1 Etiology, pp. 1139–1148. Editor: H.E. Nieburgs. Marcel Dekker, Inc., New York – Basel.

8. Ministry of Health and Welfare: *National Nutritional Survey, 1966–1980*. Department of Nutrition, Bureau of Public Health, Dai-ichi, Tokyo, Japan.

9. Hirayama, T. (1976): Metal-material workers and lung cancer in Japan: occupational carcinogenesis. *Ann. N.Y. Acad. Sci., 271*, 269.

10. Hirayama, T. (1981): Non-smoking wives of heavy smokers have a higher risk of lung cancer: a study from Japan. *Brit. med. J., 282*, 183.

11. Kim, D.S. (1968): Cancer in Korea. *Kor. J. Path., 2, Suppl.*

12. Korean Cancer Society (1976): Cancer Registry. *J. Kor. med. Ass., 19/5.*

13. Ministry of Health (1980): *Adult Disease Survey, October 11, 1979*. Seoul, Korea.

14. Jussawala, J. and Jain, D.K. (1979): Lung cancer in Greater Bombay: correlations with religion and smoking habits. *Brit. J. Cancer, 40*, 437.

15. Spencer, H. (1970): *Pathology of the Lung, 2nd ed.* Pergamon Press, London.

16. Godeau, P., De Saint-Maur, P., Herreman, G., Rault, P., Cenac, A. and Rosenthal, P. (1974): Carcinome bronchiolo-alvéolaire et sclérodermie. *Sem. Hôp. Paris, 50*, 1161.

The biology of lung cancer

Adi F. Gazdar, Desmond N. Carney and John D. Minna

Lung cancer represents a major form of cancer, both in incidence and mortality, with about 110,000 new cases in the U.S.A. every year. Only the four major forms of bronchogenic carcinoma – epidermoid, small-cell, large-cell and adenocarcinoma – accounting for about 98% of non-pleural pulmonary malignancies will be discussed. To keep the number of references to a manageable number, recent useful references will be often cited in place of multiple original works.

While the incidence of lung cancer types varies worldwide, epidermoid is the commonest. In the U.S.A., adenocarcinoma and small-cell carcinoma have approximately the same incidence, with large-cell occurring less commonly (1). With the advent of modern therapy, it became apparent that the histological type may greatly influence the clinical presentation, response to therapy and survival. Small-cell lung cancer (SCLC) stands out as a distinct entity (1, 2). It usually presents with distant metastases, occult or obvious; it is associated with a wide variety of paraneoplastic syndromes; even Stage I cases are seldom cured by surgical resection; the vast majority of cases respond dramatically to chemo- and radiotherapy; and some suitably treated patients with extensive disease survive for long periods. While there are differences in presentation, response to therapy and survival among the non-small-cell lung cancers (NSCLC), they are relatively modest. Thus, there is a tendency among clinicians to divide lung cancer into two major clinico-therapeutic categories: SCLC and NSCLC.

The large number of unique features associated with SCLC led to an intensive study of its biology. While initial progress was slow, the establishment of many well-characterized continuous cell lines, largely by two groups of investigators (3, 4), has resulted in an explosion of recent knowledge (Fig. 1). In this chapter, we review the major developments in the biology of lung cancer, and compare and contrast the properties of SCLC and NSCLC. Because comparable studies on the latter have lagged far behind those on SCLC, we seldom separate out the component types of NSCLC, but analyze them as a group.

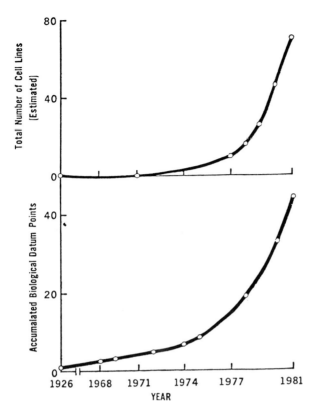

FIG. 1. *Relationship between establishment of small-cell lung cancer (SCLC) cell lines and increase in biological knowledge. The upper panel demonstrates the cumulative number (estimated) of SCLC cell lines established by various laboratories. In the lower panel, important biological discoveries about SCLC are plotted cumulatively. Clinical landmarks are not included. Approximately 50% of the biological discoveries within the last 5 years have resulted from in-vitro studies of continuous cell lines.*

Growth rate, DNA contents and chromosomal abnormalities

The rapid spread of SCLC and its responsiveness to therapy suggest a rapidly growing tumor, and initial studies appeared to confirm this belief. However, more recent, carefully conducted studies indicate that the clinical doubling times of SCLC usually exceed 2 months and are similar to those of squamous-cell and large-cell carcinomas (5). However, SCLC does have a relatively high labeling index, suggesting that rapid cell proliferation is accompanied by considerable cell death. Cell

15

culture studies (see below) confirm this concept. By contrast, adenocarcinomas have long doubling times and low labeling indices, findings that are compatible with their resistance to therapy.

Flow-cytometric studies (6) indicate that the vast majority of lung cancers have an aneuploid DNA content. Although all lung cancers have a wide range of aneuploidy and chromosome content, in general, NSCLC have a higher percentage of aneuploidy and higher DNA contents than SCLC tumors (P. Bunn and authors' unpublished data).

Chromosomal banding studies demonstrate a specific chromosomal abnormality associated with SCLC (7, 8). At least one chromosome 3 in all SCLC metaphases examined had a deletion involving the short arm. The shortest region of overlap analysis showed that the common region deleted was deletion 3p(14–23). The defect was present in all SCLC tumors, cell lines and heterotransplanted tumors, but not in other autologous cells. Thus, deletion 3p is a specific, acquired somatic defect. Of interest, SCLC cell lines that had lost their characteristic biochemical properties retained the deletion 3p. While a deletion of 3p was seen in some NSCLC metaphases, the specific 3p(14–23) deletion was not consistently found in other forms of lung cancer. Thus, the deletion 3p may be the ultimate arbitrator of whether a cell line or tumor is of SCLC lineage. Whether the deletion is the cause or only associated with the malignant behavior of SCLC remains to be determined. Similarly, whether the defect represents an absolute deletion of 3p or a translocation of 3p material to another chromosome is under investigation.

While the majority of lung cancers have a single DNA peak by flow cytometry, approximately 10–20% (9) (P. Bunn, personal communication) have two or more aneuploid peaks. These findings indicate that some tumors display clonal heterogeneity, and may have therapeutic implications (different clones may vary in sensitivity to drugs).

In-vitro clonogenic assays

In-vitro clonogenic assays for tumor 'stem' cells have been advocated as a method for drug selection (10). In general, tumor cells are disaggregated into single cells and suspended in semi-solid growth medium overlying a firmer base layer. Approximately 1 agar colony ('clone') occurs per 10^3–10^4 cells plated, and colonies are enumerated 7–21 days later. Using this technique, in-vitro sensitivity data have been generated for a large number of different human tumors (11). We have developed assays for cloning specimens from lung cancer patients (12, 13). There is an excellent correlation between the presence of tumor cells in the specimens and the formation of colonies. The cells in the colonies cytologically resemble the original tumor cells and have the same degree of aneuploidy. While attempts to propagate the colonies indefinitely by transfer to liquid media are usually unsuccessful, the 'stem' cell nature of the colonies is demonstrated by their tumorigenicity in athymic nude mice following intracranial injection (13, 14).

While the studies discussed above may be used to study the biology of lung cancer, are they of therapeutic use? The majority of tumor-containing specimens from marrow and effusions form colonies, but the success rate for solid tumors (which require considerable disaggregation) is much lower. The overall colony-forming efficiency is low (<0.001–0.1% per plated cell and 0.1–1.6% per plated tumor cell) – a major problem when few tumor cells are present in small specimens obtained during routine staging procedures. This limits the numbers and concentrations of drugs that can be tested. In addition, the low colony-forming efficiency means that only a small fraction of the tumor cell population is being tested.

How accurate are drug-testing data? For many human tumors, the negative predictions are much more accurate than the positive ones (11). We tested a number of drugs known to be active against SCLC using fresh specimens and established tumor cell lines. Using fresh SCLC specimens and correlating the data with the patients' response to therapy, the accuracy for a negative prediction was 100% and for a positive prediction 75% (15). Because of the problems of obtaining adequate numbers of colonies from tumor samples, we also tested continuous SCLC cell lines established from untreated and relapsed patients (15). The accuracy for a negative prediction was 100% and for a positive prediction 92%. Thus, continuous cell lines may be useful for predicting in-vivo response to chemotherapy and for the evaluation of new drugs. In fact, this accuracy appears great enough that clinical trials may be designed to test prospectively whether in-vitro drug selection is of clinical benefit. This appears to us to be the major new avenue to design clinical trials.

Heterotransplantation

Many human tumors, including lung cancers, can be successfully transplanted into athymic nude mice (14, 16). About 45–60% of lung cancers will form tumors after subcutaneous injection, provided adequate numbers of tumor cells are present ($>10^5$). The tumors grow progressively, but usually are non-invasive and seldom metastasize. Histologically, they closely resemble the original tumors. Intracranial injection of cells results in tumors that localize to the meninges and other intracranial sites. Intracranial tumors are locally invasive and are invariably fatal, but also do not metastasize. Because the tumor-inducing dose for intracranial tumors is 10–1000-fold less than that for subcutaneous injection, intracranial inoculation is a useful technique when small numbers of tumor cells are present. It may be a useful model for meningeal carcinomatosis, a major clinical problem associated with SCLC.

Heterotransplanted tumors are useful sources for the establishment of continuous cell lines because their success rate is higher than from fresh tumor specimens (14). In addition, heterotransplantation may be useful for determining the tumorigenicity and cell type of continuous lines and agar colonies. They are useful for growing large quantities of cells for biological or immunological studies. Currently, many heterotransplanted human tumors are being evaluated as predictors of drug sensitivity. Whether some of these will eventually replace the rodent models currently in use for drug screening remains to be determined. The most encouraging data with regard to human lung cancer come from Dr. Steel's group in the United Kingdom (49). They have compared the chemosensitivity of human SCLC and NSCLC heterotransplanted into immune deprived mice with the identical chemotherapy used to treat the patients donating the tumors. They found excellent correlation between the response in the heterotransplants and the response in the patients. This is a further indication for using a tumor cell line outside of the patient to select therapy.

Isolation of cellular transforming genes from human lung cancer

One of the most exciting new developments is the application of gene transfer technology to detect and isolate transforming genes from human lung cancer and other tumors (17). In brief, the method consists of extracting DNA from human tumors and transfecting it into nonmalignant rodent cells such as NIH/3T3. After 2 weeks, morphologically altered foci consisting of cells with loss of contact inhibition appear. These foci are picked and cloned, and yield lines capable of growth in soft agar and are tumorigenic (18–20).

The presence of human DNA in these mouse cells is confirmed by the Southern blotting technique. DNA is extracted from transformed cells, cut with different restriction endonucleases and electrophoresed in agarose gels. The DNA is then transferred by the Southern procedure to a nitrocellulose filter, and DNA bands containing human sequences detected by overlying the gel with labeled DNA containing the 'Alu' sequence of human genes. These 'Alu' sequences are arrays of highly repeated sequences scattered throughout the human genome that are distinct from any mouse sequence (21). Thus, their presence marks a human gene in a mouse cell.

18

When mouse cells transformed with human lung cancer DNA are probed, a large number of bands are seen, indicating that a large number of human genes (e.g. 100) have been stransferred. The DNA from these transformants is re-isolated and used to transform another set of mouse cells. This time, only a few human genes are found. By analyzing the bands from a number of transformants, the bands containing the putative lung cancer genes can be identified. Using similar approaches, a number of laboratories have isolated transforming genes from human breast, lung, colon bladder and neuroblastoma cell lines. Of great interest, it appears as if a human colon cancer line, an adenocarcinoma line (A549) and an SCLC line (LX-1) have donated the same transforming gene (20) (Weinberg et al., personal communication).

Following the detection of human transforming sequences, several laboratories are trying to clone the transforming genes, using recombinant DNA techniques, to prepare large amounts of specific DNA. This should allow tests of biological activity and eventual determination of the exact DNA sequence. A major unanswered question is whether all lung cancer cells will yield the same transforming genes. In any event, application of this new technology promises to revolutionize our approach to the biology of lung cancer cells.

In-vitro growth of lung cancer

With the advent of drug sensitivity testing and the isolation of genes from human tumors, the ability to reproductively grow human lung cancers from individual patients becomes extremely important. In brief, lung cancer grows well in patients, but has been difficult to grow in culture. Thus, it was important to establish techniques for culturing lung cancer cells.

Since the first report of an SCLC line more than a decade ago (22), approximately 70 continuous lines have been established (Fig. 1), predominantly by our group and the Dartmouth group (3, 4). The two groups have used somewhat different culture methods and their respective cell lines differ in growth properties. Unless otherwise stated, our remarks will apply only to lines established in our laboratory.

While early attempts to establish SCLC lines seldom were successful, with experience the majority of specimens containing adequate numbers of viable tumor cells can be established as continuous cell lines. Specimens from marrow, effusions and nude mouse heterotransplants are easier to propagate than solid tumor specimens. With the use of conditioned medium from other established SCLC lines, as well as defined serum-free medium (see below), we have established and characterized approximately 35 SCLC cell lines. In addition, using conventional techniques, we have established 12 cell lines from other pulmonary malignancies. These lines, plus additional lines provided by other investigators, provide us with a spectrum of NSCLC tumor types (squamous-cell, large-cell, adenocarcinoma, mucoepidermoid bronchogenic carcinomas as well as mesotheliomas). Thus, we can compare and contrast the properties of SCLC and NSCLC.

All cell lines are continuous, free of stromal cells, and aneuploid, and most are clonable and tumorigenic. Their DNA contents and chromosome compositions are similar to the tumors from which they were derived. The tumors they induce in nude mice are morphologically similar to the original tumors. Cytologically, the SCLC cells demonstrate the classic features of the intermediate type of SCLC, while the NSCLC lines (other than mucin-secreting adenocarcinomas) appear undifferentiated, and electron microscopy or histological examination of heterotransplanted tumors is required for further identification.

Major differences exist between the growth properties of SCLC and NSCLC lines. SCLC lines replicate as tight or loose cell aggregates, while NSCLC lines demonstrate substrate adhesion (as do most human epithelial tumors). The SCLC lines have long population-doubling times. Cytological examination reveals many mitoses and many necrotic cells. Thus, as with SCLC tumors, short cell-cycle times accompanied by considerable cell death result in a long population-doubling time. By

TABLE 1. *Differences in properties of small-cell lung cancer (SCLC) and non-small-cell lung cancer (NSCLC) cell lines*

Property	SCLC	NSCLC
Substrate adherence	absent	present
Doubling time	long	relatively short
Cloning efficiency	low	relatively high
Aneuploidy	present	present
Deletion 3p(14–23)	present	absent
Tumorigenicity	yes	yes
L-dopa decarboxylase	high specific activity	low or absent
Neuron-specific enolase	high specific activity	low or absent
Dense core 'neurosecretory' granules	present	absent
Bombesin	present	absent
Other peptide hormones (e.g. ACTH, AVP, calcitonin)	often present	occasionally present
Creatine kinase (CK) and CK-BB	high specific activity	low
SCLC antigen (monoclonal antibody defined)	present	absent

20

contrast, NSCLC lines have relatively fast doubling times and lack significant cell necrosis. SCLC lines have low cloning efficiencies, while NSCLC lines clone much more efficiently (3). Unlike colonies obtained from fresh lung tumor specimens, clones of SCLC and NSCLC cell lines can usually be propagated to mass culture. The differences in biological properties between SCLC and NSCLC lines are summarized in Table 1.

Growth of lung cancers in defined media

The use of defined media for the growth of specific cell types (23) has greatly advanced our knowledge of cell biology. The advantages of defined media include: (1) identification of specific growth factors; (2) selective growth of differentiated normal and malignant cells; (3) a method for in-vitro growth of some cells and tumors that do not replicate in conventional serum-supplemented media; and (4) ease of isolation and analysis of secreted cellular products. Our initial studies indicated that the majority of SCLC lines replicate in RPMI-1640 medium supplemented with hydrocortisone, insulin, transferrin and 17β-estradiol (HITES medium) (24). HITES medium is selective for SCLC and it does not support the efficient replication of NSCLC cells. In addition, over 90% of SCLC tumor specimens selectively replicate in HITES (25), a higher percentage than in serum-supplemented medium. SCLC lines established and maintained in HITES medium retain the characteristic morphological and biological properties of other SCLC lines.

While HITES medium has proved to be effective for establishing and maintaining SCLC cultures, there are indications that it is an incomplete medium: (1) some SCLC tumors and cell lines replicate very slowly in HITES; (2) tumor specimens and cell lines rarely clone in HITES; and (3) addition of conditioned medium from an established SCLC line (NCI-N592) to HITES enhances SCLC growth and clonogenicity. Thus, we investigated the effects of other additions to HITES medium. We have found that the addition of arginine vasopressin (AVP), bovine serum albumin, bombesin and a combination of ethanolamine/phosphoethanolamine to HITES (SCLC-2 medium) enhances SCLC growth and clonogenicity (26). These observations are of additional interest because AVP and bombesin are SCLC tumor products (see below); they may well represent examples of autocrine secretion (i.e. a tumor product that stimulates the tumor's growth). It is possible that manipulation of AVP and bombesin could be used as new therapeutic strategies for inhibiting SCLC growth.

Our studies with defining media for NSCLC are at an embryonic stage. Currently, we are testing an incomplete medium that partially supports the growth of some lung adenocarcinomas (27).

Monoclonal antibodies

The somatic cell hybridization techniques developed by Kohler and Milstein (28) for preparing monoclonal antibodies have been used widely to isolate highly specific antibodies including those directed against tumor cell surface antigens. We have used similar methods to generate monoclonal antibodies with specificity for human lung cancers (29, 30). We immunized mice and rats with SCLC cell lines and fused the spleens from immunized rodents with a continuous mouse myeloma cell line. Culture fluids of the resultant hybrid cells were screened for antibody activity against a panel of SCLC cells as well as other autologous cells from the same patients. Antibodies that reacted with the former, but not the latter, were selected, cloned repeatedly and tested against a large panel of human and other species cell lines, both normal and neoplastic. Using sensitive radioimmune assays, we found that many of these antibodies reacted with many different SCLC tumors and cell lines, but not with normal liver, lung, skin fibroblasts or B lymphoblastoid cells. Most of the antibodies react with human neuroblastoma and breast cell lines.

Of two highly characterized antibodies, one of mouse origin (534F8) crossreacts with some NSCLC lines, while another (604A9) of rat origin is highly specific for SCLC. Thus, different types of lung cancer may share certain antigens as well as express specific antigens. In addition to reacting with cell lines, the antibodies reacted with SCLC autopsy material and bone marrow metastases. Some of the antibodies are cytotoxic for SCLC cells when incubated with complement and also inhibit clonal growth of the cells. In collaboration with Dr. Paul Bunn, using a fluorescent activated cell sorter (FACS), we found that the percentage of antigen-positive cells in SCLC lines varied from 10 to 90%. Thus, the cells of individual cell lines demonstrate a varying degree of heterogeneity of antigen expression. Using a panel of different antibodies, we are currently using immunohistochemical methods to study antigenic patterns of a large number of various types of lung cancer.

Monoclonal antibodies to tumor cells have major potential clinical applications (30) including: (1) detection of circulating antigen or antibody; (2) detection of small numbers of tumor cells at metastatic sites; (3) use of isotope-labeled antibodies for nuclear scanning; (4) therapeutic uses using antibody conjugated with drugs, toxins or specific delivery systems. At present, there is considerable interest in using autologous bone marrow transplants to 'rescue' SCLC patients from otherwise lethal doses of chemotherapy. Because the marrow is a favorite site for occult or detectable metastases, monoclonal antibodies may be used to eliminate tumor cells ex vivo, prior to marrow reinfusion. Some of these applications, already in use with other tumor types (31), will be tried in lung cancer in the near future.

Endocrine properties of small-cell lung cancer

SCLC is frequently associated with polypeptide hormone secretion in vivo and in vitro (32, 33). While hormone secretion by SCLC was initially regarded as 'ectopic', we have gradually realized that SCLC (and perhaps carcinoids) are tumors of endocrine cells and arise from, or are closely related to, similar endocrine (Kulchitsky) cells present in small numbers in the normal tracheobronchial tree (34, 35).

Pearse identified a widely distributed system of cells having amine precursor uptake and decarboxylation (APUD) properties (36). While a number of properties have been attributed to APUD cells, the most important and consistent of these are: (1) amine precursor uptake; (2) decarboxylation of precursor to 'biogenic' amine product by a specific enzyme, L-dopa decarboxylase (DDC); (3) amine or polypeptide product; (4) storage of products in cytoplasmic, membrane-bound, dense core ('neurosecretory') granules; and (5) presence of a special isoenzyme of the glycolytic enzyme enolase, neuron-specific enolase (NSE). SCLC tumors and cell lines express all of the classic APUD cell properties (3, 37–38). In fact, the levels of DDC and NSE in SCLC are the highest we have detected in any form of tumor. These properties are seldom expressed in NSCLC (Fig. 2).

While many peptides may be produced by SCLC, their concentrations usually are low, and there is considerable clonal variation in expression (39). By contrast, we have recently shown that the small peptide, bombesin, is expressed in all SCLC lines and tumors (40) at very high concentrations, and that its expression is retained in all SCLC clones examined. Bombesin is present in pulmonary endocrine cells, especially during fetal and neonatal life (41). Because of this, we have proposed that SCLC arises from a 'bombesinergic' subset of the pulmonary endocrine cells (40).

Other differences between lung cancers

We have reported major differences in the intracellular concentrations of creatine kinase (CK) and its BB isoenzyme (CK-BB) between SCLC and NSCLC (42). CK is an enzyme present in all cells and it exists in 3 isomeric forms: BB (brain form), MM (muscle form) and MB (hybrid form). Normal lung and NSCLC tumors and cell lines have low concentrations of CK, while SCLC tumors and lines have exceedingly high concentrations (up to 3.5% of the soluble protein). In normal lung and in all lung cancers, the major CK isoenzyme is CK-BB. Thus, CK levels in SCLC are quantitatively, but not qualitatively, different from those of normal lung and NSCLC. In SCLC, there is a constant ratio between

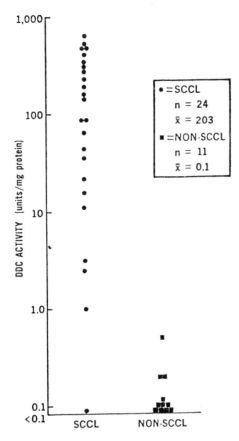

FIG. 2. *L-dopa decarboxylase (DDC) concentrations in lung cancer cell lines. Values for small-cell carcinoma (SCCL) are displayed in the left-hand column and those for other forms of lung cancer in the right-hand column. DDC concentrations were measured enzymatically and are expressed as units/mg soluble protein. Note log scale.*

the concentrations of enzymatic CK and immunoreactive CK-BB, indicating that a constant proportion (or all) of the CK-BB is functional. Because CK and its substrate, creatine, act as a source for the rapid regeneration of ATP during active metabolism, these findings suggest that the energy requirements of SCLC are very different from those of normal lung and NSCLC. Major differences exist between SCLC and NSCLC in their patterns of expression of membrane receptors for peptide growth factors (43). NSCLC (and most other epithelial cells and tumors) have receptors for epidermal growth factor, while they are lacking in SCLC. By contrast, certain SCLC (but not NSCLC) tumors express receptors for nerve growth factor, which are expressed by relatively few tumors (some neural tumors and melanomas).

Drs. Stephen Baylin and Joel Shaper, in collaboration with us, have studied the cell surface protein phenotypes of the major forms of lung cancer (44). SCLC is characterized by the presence of 12 unique proteins (molecular weight 40–80 kD) and the absence of proteins >100 kD. The NSCLC tumors have phenotypes similar to each other, including the presence of 5 proteins of >100 kD and 8 smaller proteins not present in SCLC. Of interest, the surface protein phenotype of SCLC is closer to that of human neuroblastoma than NSCLC – further evidence that the former is a neuroendocrine cell. Surface proteins may provide markers for studying further the cell lineages involved in the formation of normal and neoplastic bronchial epithelium.

New clinical markers

This is not the forum for an extensive review of the many substances reported as potential clinical markers for lung cancer. Because SCLC may secrete many polypeptide hormones and other substances, more markers have been associated with it (32) than NSCLC. The properties of an ideal clinical marker include: (1) high intracellular levels in all, or almost all, tumors and little or no heterogeneity within individual tumors; (2) it is actively secreted by tumor cells into the blood or body fluids; (3) the substance is stable in blood and other fluids; (4) detectable blood levels are seldom present with other tumors or disease states; (5) a relatively simple, inexpensive, highly sensitive assay is available.

At present, none of the known markers fulfil all these criteria, even for SCLC. The most important difficulty is the heterogeneity of marker expression within individual tumors. Some of the intracellular markers we have investigated (DDC, NSE, CK, CK-BB, bombesin) are present in high concentrations in virtually all classic SCLC tumors. While some of these substances have potential as clinical markers, none is an ideal marker. DDC is measured by a relatively insensitive enzymatic assay, and we have not detected measurable blood levels in any SCLC patient. CK levels are elevated in many disease states. CK-BB and NSE have low background levels; elevated levels are present in many patients with extensive disease, but drop to normal during remission (42) (D.N.C., M. Zweig, P. Marangos and A.F.G., unpublished data). They are not actively secreted by tumor cells, but are released by dying and dead cells. They are useful markers for tumor bulk and response to therapy, but are not useful for the detection of early tumors. Bombesin is actively secreted by SCLC cells; unfortunately, it is destroyed by protease present in RBCs and other tissues. Bombesin assays are technically difficult and blood samples require special handling. While we are in the midst of a prospective study, our preliminary data indicate that plasma bombesin levels may be another marker of tumor bulk (T. Moody, C. Pert, and authors' unpublished data). While we have many excellent intracellular markers for SCLC, the search for an ideal clinical marker continues.

Lung cancer interconversions and interrelationships

It is apparent that SCLC is very different from other lung carcinomas. Pearse (36) originally postulated that all APUD cells had a neuroepithelial origin (and thus SCLC would have a different origin from the rest of the endodermally derived bronchial mucosa and NSCLC). While this theory originally had considerable appeal, further evidence has made the concept of a separate origin for SCLC untenable (34). One important piece of evidence that all lung cancers have a common origin is the histological interrelationships of lung cancers. About 6% of SCLC tumors have other large cell types at presentation, while at autopsy about 35% of SCLC tumors have other histological types of lung cancer, or have completely converted to an NSCLC morphology (45). Similar changes occur in vitro (34). For example, morphological change from a small-cell to a large-cell variant is accompanied by loss of many of the characteristic markers of SCLC such as dense core granules, L-DDC, peptide hormone production, and monoclonal antibody binding. However, the characteristic cytological marker deletion 3p is retained (34, 46). In addition, clonal studies indicate that both components of adenosquamous carcinomas are derived from a common stem cell (47). On occasion, non-endocrine lung tumors may express endocrine properties (48).

The morphological and biochemical studies cited above strongly indicate that the spectrum of lung cancers represents neoplastic changes within a common cell lineage (48). Because of this, we currently regard epidermoid, adenocarcinoma and SCLC as 'differentiated' tumors (34), while large-cell carcinoma consists of a heterogeneous group including: (1) poorly differentiated tumors; (2) true undifferentiated (potentially stem cell) tumors; (3) previously differentiated tumors that have 'lost' their differentiated properties. The use of cytogenetic and other markers preserved in these undifferentiated forms of lung cancer should be of use in sorting out the various patterns of tumor cell differentiation.

Concluding remarks

Knowledge of the biology of lung cancer has major potential clinical applications including: (1) prevention; (2) early diagnosis and staging; (3) selection of therapy; (4) monitoring response to therapy; and (5) newer therapeutic approaches, such as hormonal manipulation of tumors or targeting of therapy with monoclonal antibodies. Lung cancers represent a spectrum of tumor types sharing certain properties and probably a common stem cell of origin. Clinically and biologically, they fall into two broad groups – SCLC and NSCLC. Major strides have been made recently in our understanding of the biology of SCLC, following intensive study of many established cell lines. Knowledge about other forms of lung cancer has accumulated at a much slower rate, in part because of the diverse nature of NSCLC, and from a lack of sufficient in-vitro systems. These deficiencies are slowly being corrected and NSCLC will soon receive the same in-depth study as SCLC. Hopefully, we will see the clinical implementation of these cell-biological findings in the near future.

References

1. Minna, J.D., Higgins, G.A. and Glatstein, E.J. (1982): Cancer of the lung. In: *Principles and Practice of Oncology,* pp. 396–473. Editors: V.T. DeVita, S. Hellman and S.A. Rosenberg. J. Lippincott, Philadelphia.
2. Cohen, M.H. and Matthews, M.J. (1978): Small cell bronchogenic carcinoma: a distinct clinicopathologic entity. *Semin. Oncol., 5,* 234–243.
3. Gazdar, A.F., Carney, D.N., Russell, E.K., Sims, H.L., Baylin, S.B., Bunn, P.A., Guccion, J.G. and Minna, J.D. (1980): Establishment of continuous, clonable cultures of small cell carcinoma of the lung which have amine precursor uptake and decarboxylation properties. *Cancer Res., 40,* 3502–3507.
4. Pettengill, O.S., Sorenson, G.D., Wurster-Hill, D.H., Curphey, T.J., Nou, W.W., Cate, C.C. and Maurer, L.H. (1980): Isolation and growth characteristics of continuous cell lines from small-cell carcinoma of the lung. *Cancer, 45,* 906–918.
5. Shackney, S.E., Straus, M.J. and Bunn, P.A. (1981): The growth characteristics of small cell carcinoma of the lung. In: *Small Cell Lung Cancer*, pp. 225–234. Editors: F.A. Greco, R.K. Oldham and P.A. Bunn. Grune and Stratton, New York.
6. Barlogie, B., Drewinko, B., Schumann, J., Gohde, W., Doskik, G., Latreille, J., Johnston, D.A. and Freireich, E.J. (1980): Cellular DNA content as a marker of neoplasia in man. *Amer. J. Med., 69,* 195–203.
7. Whang-Peng, J., Kao-Shan, C.S., Lee, E.C., Bunn, P.A., Carney, D.N., Gazdar, A.F. and Minna, J.D. (1982): Specific chromosome defect associated with human small-cell lung cancer: deletion 3p(14–23). *Science, 215,* 181–182.
8. Whang-Peng, J.W., Bunn, P.A., Kao-Shan, C.S., Carney, D.N., Minna, J.D. and Gazdar, A.F. (1982): A non-random chromosomal abnormality,

del 3p(14–23) in human small cell lung cancer. *Cancer Gen. Cytogen.*, in press.

9. Vindelov, L.L., Hansen, H.H., Christensen, H.I., Spang-Thomsen, M., Hirsch, F.R., Hansen, M. and Nissen, N.I. (1980): Clonal heterogeneity of small-cell anaplastic carcinoma of the lung demonstrated by flow-cytometric DNA analysis. *Cancer Res. 40*, 4295–4300.

10. Salmon, S.E., Hamburger, A.W., Soehnlen, B., Durie, B.G., Alberts, D.S. and Moon, T.E. (1978): Quantitation of differential sensitivity of human tumor stem cells to anticancer drugs. *New Engl. J. Med., 298*, 1321–1327.

11. Von Hoff, D.D., Casper, J., Bradley, E., Sandback, J., Jones, D. and Makuch, R. (1981): Association between human tumor colony-forming assay results and response of an individual patient's tumor to chemotherapy. *Amer. J. Med., 70*, 1027–1032.

12. Carney, D.N., Gazdar, A.F. and Minna, J.D. (1980): Positive correlation between histologic tumor involvement and generation of tumor cell colonies in agarose in specimens taken directly from patients with small cell carcinoma of the lung. *Cancer Res., 40*, 1820–1823.

13. Carney, D.N., Gazdar, A.F., Bunn, P.A. and Guccion, J.G. (1982): Demonstration of the stem cell nature of clonogenic tumor cells from lung cancer patients. *Stem Cells*, in press.

14. Gazdar, A.F., Carney, D.N., Sims, H.L. and Simmons, A. (1981): Heterotransplantation of small cell carcinoma of the lung into nude mice: comparison of intracranial and subcutaneous routes. *Int. J. Cancer*, in press.

15. Carney, D.N., Gazdar, A.F. and Minna, J.D. (1982): In vitro chemosensitivity of clinical specimens and cell lines of small cell lung cancer. *Proc. ASCO/AACR*, in press.

16. Shimosato, Y., Kameya, T., Nagai, K., Hirohashi, S., Koide, T., Hayashi, H. and Nomura, T. (1976): Transplantation in human tumors into nude mice. *J. nat. Cancer Inst., 56*, 1251–1260.

17. Rigby, P.W.J. (1981): The detection of cellular transforming genes. *Nature (Lond.), 290*, 186–187.

18. Shih, C., Padhy, L.C., Murrary, M. and Weinberg, R.A. (1981): Transforming genes of carcinomas and neuroblastomas introduced into mouse fibroblasts. *Nature (Lond.), 290*, 261–264.

19. Murrary, M.J., Shilo, B., Shih, C., Cowing, D., Hsu, H.W. and Weinberg, R.A. (1981): Three different human tumor cell lines contain different oncogenes. *Cell, 25*, 355–361.

20. Perucho, M., Goldfarb, M., Shimizu, K., Lama, C., Fogh, J. and Wigler, M. (1982): Common and different transforming genes are contained in human tumor derived cell lines. *Cell*, in press.

21. Rinehart, F.P., Ritch, T.G., Deininger, P.L. and Schmid, C.W. (1981): Renaturation rate studies of a single family of interspersed repeated sequences in human DNA. *Biochemistry, 20*, 3003–3010.

22. Oboshi, S., Tsugawa, S., Seido, T., Shimosato, Y., Koide, T. and Ishikawa, S. (1971): A new floating cell line derived from human pulmonary carcinoma of oat cell type. *Gann, 62*, 505–514.

23. Barnes, D. and Sato, G. (1980): Methods for growth of cultured cells in serum-free medium. *Analyt. Biochem., 102*, 255–270.

24. Simms, E., Gazdar, A.F., Abrams, P.G. and Minna, J.D. (1980): Growth of human small cell (oat cell) carcinoma of the lung in serum-free growth factor supplemented medium. *Cancer Res., 40*, 4356–4361.

25. Carney, D.N., Bunn, P.A., Gazdar, A.F., Pagan, J.A. and Minna, J.D. (1981): Selective growth of small cell carcinoma of the lung obtained from patient biopsies in serum-free hormone supplemented medium. *Proc. nat. Acad. Sci., 78*, 3185–3189.

26. Oie, H.K., Carney, D.N., Gazdar, A.F. and Minna, J.D. (1982): Soft agarose cloning of small cell lung carcinoma in serum-free defined medium. *Proc. ASCO/AACR*, in press.

27. Brower, M., Carney, D., Oie, H., Matthews, M. and Minna, J. (1982): Growth of human adenocarcinoma of the lung cell lines and clinical specimens in serum-free defined medium. *Proc. ASCO/AACR*, in press.

28. Kohler, G. and Milstein, C. (1975): Continuous cultures of fused cells secreting antibody of predestined specificity. *Nature (Lond.), 256*, 495–497.

29. Cuttitta, F., Rosen, S., Gazdar, A.F. and Minna, J.D. (1981): Monoclonal antibodies which demonstrate specificity for several types of human lung cancer. *Proc. nat. Acad. Sci., 78*, 4591–4595.

30. Minna, J.D., Cuttitta, F., Rosen, S., Bunn, P.A., Carney, D.N., Gazdar, A.F. and Krasnow, S. (1982): Methods for production of monoclonal antibodies with specificity for human lung cancer cells. *In Vitro*, 1058–1070.

31. Miller, R.A. and Levy, R. (1981): In vivo effects of murine hybridoma monoclonal antibody in human T cell neoplasms. *Clin. Res., 29*, 529A.

32. Greco, F.A., Hainsworth, J., Sismani, A., Richardson, R.L., Hande, K.R. and Oldham, R.K. (1981): Hormone production and paraneoplastic syndromes. In: *Small Cell Lung Cancer*, pp. 177–233. Editors: F.A. Greco, R.K. Oldham and P.A. Bunn. Grune and Stratton, New York.

33. Sorenson, G.D., Pettengill, O.S., Brinck-Johnsen, T., Cate, C.C. and Maurer, L.H. (1981): Hormone production by cultures of small cell carcinoma of the lung. *Cancer, 47*, 1289–1296.

34. Gazdar, A.F., Carney, D.N., Guccion, J.G. and Baylin, S.B. (1981): Small cell carcinoma of the lung: cellular origin and relationship to other pulmonary tumors. In: *Small Cell Lung Cancer*, pp. 145–175. Editors: R.K. Oldman and P.A. Bunn. Grune and Stratton, New York.

35. Becker, K.L. and Gazdar, A.F. (1982): The pulmonary endocrine cell and the tumors to which it gives rise. In: *Comparative Respiratory Tract Carcinogenesis*. Editor: H. Reznik-Schuller. CRC Press, New York. In press.

36. Pearse, A.G. (1969): The cytochemistry and ultrastructure of polypeptide hormone-producing cells of the APUD system and the embryologic, physiologic and pathologic implications of the concept. *J. Histochem. Cytochem., 17*, 303–313.

37. Baylin, S.B., Abeloff, M.D., Goodwin, G., Carney, D.N. and Gazdar, A.F. (1980): Activities of L-dopa decarboxylase and diamine oxidase (histaminase) in lung cancers and decarboxylase as a marker for small (oat) cell

cancer in culture. *Cancer Res., 40*, 1990–1994.

38. Marangos, P.J., Gazdar, A.F. and Carney, D.N. (1982): Neuron specific enolase in human small cell carcinoma cultures. *Cancer Lett.,* in press.

39. Radice, P.A. and Dermody, W.C. (1980): Clonal heterogeneity of hormone production by continuous cultures of small cell carcinoma of the lung. *Proc. ASCO/AACR, 21,* 41.

40. Moody, T.W., Pert, C.B., Gazdar, A.F., Carney, D.N. and Minna, J.D. (1981): High levels of intracellular bombesin characterize human small-cell lung carcinoma. *Science, 214,* 1246–1248.

41. Wharton, J., Polak, J.M., Bloom, S.R. and Pearse, A.G. (1978): Bombesin-like immunoreactivity in the lung. *Nature (Lond.), 273,* 769–770.

42. Gazdar, A.F., Zweig, M.H., Carney, D.N., Van Steirteghen, A.C., Baylin, S.B. and Minna, J.D. (1981): Levels of creatine kinase and its BB isoenzyme in lung cancer tumors and cultures. *Cancer Res., 41,* 2773–2777.

43. Sherwin, S.A., Minna, J.D., Gazdar, A.F. and Todaro, G.J. (1981): Expression of epidermal and nerve growth factor receptors and soft agar growth factor production by human lung cancer cells. *Cancer Res., 41,* 3538–3542.

44. Baylin, S.B., Gazdar, A.F., Minna, J.D. and Shaper, J.H. (1982): The cell surface protein phenotype distinguishes between the major forms of human lung cancer in culture. Submitted for publication.

45. Matthews, M.J. and Gazdar, A.F. (1981): Pathology of small cell carcinoma of the lung and its subtypes: a clinicopathological correlation. In: *Lung Cancer,* pp. 283–306. Editor: R.B. Livingston. Martinus Nijhoff, Boston, MS.

46. Abeloff, M.D., Eggleston, J.C., Mendelsohn, G., Ettinger, D. and Baylin, S.B. (1979): Changes in morphologic and biochemical characteristics of small cell carcinoma of the lung. *Amer. J. Med., 66,* 757–764.

47. Steele, V.E. and Netteshein, P. (1981): Unstable cellular differentiation in adenosquamous cell carcinoma. *J. nat. Cancer Inst., 67,* 149–154.

48. Baylin, S.B. and Gazdar, A.F. (1981): Endocrine biochemistry in the spectrum of human lung cancer: implications for the cellular origin of small cell carcinoma. In: *Small Cell Lung Cancer,* pp. 123–143. Editors: F.A. Greco, R.K. Oldham and P.A. Bunn. Grune and Stratton, New York.

49. Shorthouse, A.J., Peckham, M.J., Smyth, J.F. and Steel, G.G. (1980): The therapeutic response of bronchial carcinoma xenografts: a direct patient-xenograft comparison. *Brit. J. Cancer, 41, Suppl. IV,* 142–145.

Management of small-cell anaplastic carcinoma, 1980–1982

Heine H. Hansen

At the II World Congress on Lung Cancer in 1980, a review was presented on the management of small-cell carcinoma of the lung (27), focusing on staging and therapy. The purpose of the present article is to give an updated report based on data since accumulated in the literature.

The literature has been characterized in the last two years by a number of excellent review articles, dealing with all types of lung cancer, but particularly with small-cell carcinoma (6, 11, 36, 38, 40, 41, 45, 50, 51, 58, 70, 74). The number of original articles with information on possible advances in overall management has been more limited. On the other hand, several articles or abstracts covering basic aspects of the biology of small-cell carcinoma have been published recently, indicating a dynamic development in this area. Hopefully, this expansion will inspire further progress in the treatment of this disease entity in the years to come.

Of the new biological information on small-cell carcinoma it is noteworthy to mention:

1. Clonogenic assays of small-cell carcinoma have been established at several centers. It is expected that these assays will be useful for screening purposes in the selection of new compounds for clinical testing.
2. In-vitro cultures of small-cell carcinoma have been performed, giving options for further investigations of the characteristics of drug resistance at the cellular level and for the development of monoclonal antibodies (9, 14).
3. The endocrine activity of small-cell carcinoma has been characterized further, both in vitro and in vivo. Investigations using endocrine biochemistry have provided further support to the concept that small-cell anaplastic carcinoma is an APUD-tumor (5). A number of additional endocrine substances have been identified related to this tumor type, of which some (e.g. a bombesin and neurophysin) may be specific for small-cell carcinoma (56).
4. A number of different cell-lines from untreated and treated patients with small-cell anaplastic carcinoma have been transplanted to nude mice, giving options for further characterization, e.g., of the special

31

growth pattern of small-cell carcinoma, including the various subtypes (66). The system may also be useful in the development of programs for preclinical drug testing.

5. Cell-kinetic studies with flow cytometry have added considerably to our knowledge of the growth pattern of small-cell anaplastic carcinoma, both before and during therapy, the results suggesting that small-cell anaplastic carcinoma is largely a heterogeneous tumor (3, 71). Techniques are now available for continuous flow-cytometric DNA analysis during treatment of small-cell anaplastic carcinoma, making it possible to correlate the treatment with the specific cell-kinetic pattern of the individual tumor (72).

Considerable information has therefore been added to our knowledge of the biology of small-cell carcinoma, including its cellular origin and its relation to other types of lung cancer. More recent clinical-histopathological studies have further elucidated the latter point, providing important therapeutic implications.

The WHO's classification of lung tumors continues to be used with increasing frequency at major centers and by cooperative groups, thereby optimizing the possibilities for comparison of treatment results.

Several studies have emphasized that, using strictly defined criteria, small-cell anaplastic carcinoma is a distinct histopathological type which can be reproduced by different observers in more than 90% of cases (33). The remaining 10% appear to be tumors showing transitional features of other poorly differentiated lung tumors.

With regard to morphological subtyping, according to the WHO classification of 1967 and 1977, a high reproducibility of about 90% can be obtained for the individual pathologist (33). However, the criteria are not strictly enough defined for an acceptable high reproducibility among different observers, which might explain the conflicting clinical results reported in the literature using these classifications (8, 10, 16, 17, 26).

Some of the larger studies indicate that there is no clinical importance in the morphological subtyping of small-cell carcinoma when using the criteria defined by WHO (8, 26). More recently published investigations report further that the special subgroup of patients with small-cell carcinoma of the intermediate type with large-cell features has a shorter survival and a lower response rate than patients with 'pure' small-cell carcinoma (34, 47). These observations may indicate that patients with tumors containing large-cell components should be evaluated as a separate group.

At present, additional diagnostic modalities such as electron microscopy, immune histochemistry, mononclonal antibodies and DNA flow-cytometry have to be used investigationally for further characterization of the different morphological subtypes to give more consistent criteria for subtyping.

With regard to prognostic features, the stage of the disease and the performance status remain the two major features influencing the prognosis.

More recent data have indicated that a pre-treatment weight loss of >3 kg is also a significant adverse symptom. Furthermore, patients aged 60–70 years have a worse prognosis than younger patients, and males have a worse prognosis than females (77). These analyses are based, however, on univariate analyses; multivariate analyses are awaited to give more precise information on the impact of these variables on performance status.

Staging

The system first proposed by the VA Lung Cancer Study Group remains the most widely used for staging patients with small-cell anaplastic carcinoma. The VA Lung Group characterized patients as having either 'limited disease', defined as tumor confined to one hemithorax, with or without local extension, and including mediastinal adenopathy, with or without ipsilateral supraclavicular nodes, or 'extensive disease', which was defined as disease with tumor beyond these limits. The staging system was originally proposed because of its suitability for radiotherapy, the main modality of non-surgical therapy at the time when this system was introduced. In untreated patients and in patients receiving intensive chemotherapy, with or without radiotherapy, survival has been found to be significantly better for patients classified as having 'limited disease' compared to patients with 'extensive disease'. At a recent workshop meeting arranged by the IASLC, it was proposed that patients with bilateral supraclavicular nodes should also be included in the 'limited disease' category.

The use of the TNM system otherwise used for lung cancer has been less suitable for small-cell carcinoma, because 85% of the patients will be classified as having Stage III disease at the time of diagnosis.

It should be stressed that none of the above-mentioned staging systems defines the necessary number of procedures or definitions for interpretation of the different staging procedures. The development of new methods may therefore change the allocation of patients to the different stages and thereby also indirectly affect the therapeutic results, e.g. by allocating a larger percentage of patients to the group with distant metastases if extensive staging with invasive procedures is applied.

For small-cell carcinoma, the staging procedures have focused on both intrathoracic spread and extrathoracic metastatic spread. In general, it is recommended that the procedures applied should be as sensitive and specific as possible. The procedures used to detect metastatic spread often vary, however, among different investigators according to the availability of techniques, the expense of the procedures and the therapeutic implications attached to the staging. In addition, the cost, time consumption, risk, compliance of the patients and cooperation with other specialties will also influence the practical possibilities of performing the various staging procedures.

An overall view of the staging procedures most frequently used in small-cell carcinoma is given in Tables 1 and 2, with an attempt to indicate whether the procedures are considered mandatory for use as a routine screening procedure, recommended in special clinical situations, or still have to be considered as experimental.

In evaluation of intrathoracic spread, an ordinary chest X-ray still remains the most important procedure in addition to bronchoscopy.

For examination of mediastinal and intraparenchymal pulmonary masses, computerized tomograms (CT scans) are often more sensitive than conventional radiographs. Recent data by Harper and colleagues (30) indicate that, with CT scanning, spread of the primary tumor can be found to be far more extensive than when patients are evaluated by conventional X-ray. Of 35 patients conventionally staged as having localized T_1 and T_2 tumors, 27 (77%) had their stage increased to extensive T_3 disease. Similarly, subcarinal lymph nodes were found in only one patient using conventional X-ray, but in 16 patients following CT scan. Overall, 37 patients (74%) were found to have Stage III tumors by conventional staging and 47 patients (94%) using CT scanning. The authors conclude that CT scanning demonstrates the degree of intrathoracic spread far better than conventional radiology.

For confirmation of pleural involvement, thoracocentesis with cytological evaluation is the first procedure which should be performed to show whether a pleural effusion is caused by malignant spread. In addition, thoracoscopy with direct visualization and biopsy of pleural lesions is valuable in cases where the first two procedures do not give a definitive answer. For lesions in the lung parenchyma, either transbronchial biopsy or percutaneous fine-needle lung biopsy is useful to demonstrate the exact nature of a radiographic lesion.

Fiberoptic bronchoscopy has recently been utilized with increased frequency at several centers. It has been particularly useful in identifying a group of patients in apparent complete remission as shown by chest X-ray, who have residual endobronchial tumor.

Mediastinoscopy remains a valuable procedure, particularly in restaging of patients before discontinuation of therapy.

With regard to radionuclide scanning, a recent publication (54)

TABLE 1. *Staging procedures in small-cell carcinoma: intrathoracic*

	Routine screening	Symptomatic patients or special clinical indications	Experi-mental
Chest X-ray	x		
Chest tomograms		x	
Computed tomography			x
Thoracocentesis ı fluid cytology		x	
Pleural biopsy		x	
Thoracoscopy		x	
Fiberoptic bronchoscopy		x	
Mediastinoscopy		x	
^{67}Ga scan		x	

TABLE 2. *Staging procedures in small-cell carcinoma: extrathoracic sites*

	Routine screening	Symptomatic patients or special clinical indications	Experi-mental
Hepatic metastases			
Biochemical liver function tests	x		
Peritoneoscopy with liver biopsy		x	
Ultrasound examination of liver with fine-needle aspiration			x
Computed tomography of liver			x
Radionuclide liver scan		x	
Bone metastases			
Peripheral blood examination	x		
Bone marrow aspiration biopsy	x		
Radionuclide bone scan		x	
Skeletal X-rays		x	
CNS metastases			
Radionuclide brain scan		x	
Computed tomography of brain		x	
Lumbar puncture with cytological examination		x	
Lumbar puncture with evaluation of 'ectopic hormones'			x
Myelogram		x	
Other sites			
Computed tomography of abdomen			x
Whole-body ^{67}Ga scan			x

reports the superiority of ^{57}Co-bleomycin scintigraphy in the evaluation of the malignant nature of peripheral lesions on chest X-ray, and in the evaluation of hilar and mediastinal involvement, compared to scintigraphy with ^{67}Ga. However, at present, the usefulness of both ^{67}Ga and ^{57}Co-bleomycin in assessing the response of intrathoracic small-cell anaplastic carcinoma remains to be established.

In screening for liver metastases, serum alkaline phosphatase, glutamic oxaloacetic transaminase and lactic dehydrogenase remain important diagnostic tools. Radioisotope liver scintigraphy with ^{99m}Tc-sulfate is an unspecific method, and the changes observed cannot be distinguished clearly from non-malignant findings. Accordingly, other methods have to be recommended for detection of liver metastases, including peritoneoscopy with liver biopsy and ultrasound evaluation with fine-needle aspiration. Of the latter methods, peritoneoscopy with liver biopsy has for years been a well-established method in small-cell carcinoma, whereas the other methods are still under investigation. Preliminary data have indicated that CT scanning in the evaluation of 66 newly diagnosed patients with small-cell carcinoma had a sensitivity of 64% and a specificity of 92% (35). The procedure, however, demands an experienced operator and high-cost equipment which limit its general applicability.

For detection of bone metastases, bone marrow aspiration and biopsy remain the most important procedures, in addition to hematological and biochemical evaluation. It is now well documented that radiological examination of the osseous system should not be used as a routine procedure in the detection of bone metastases in small-cell carcinoma. Radionuclide bone scan remains a sensitive procedure, and it can be used as an additional procedure to bone marrow examination. However, it is recommended that abnormal findings on a bone scan should be investigated for malignancy by biopsy, before accepting an abnormal bone scan as an indicator of a metastatic lesion.

In the detection of CNS metastases, CT scanning has emerged as the best technique, being far superior to radionuclide brain scan and electroencephalograms. The specificity and sensitivity of the CT scan remains to be determined before the method can be applied as a routine screening procedure in the staging of all patients with small-cell carcinoma. Radionuclide brain scan has been found to be less sensitive than clinical examination carried out by an experienced neurologist, especially when metastases are located in the posterior cranial fossa (32).

Carcinomatous meningitis is best documented by cytological examination of the cerebrospinal fluid, but myelography is also valuable (2). The value of lumbar puncture as a screening procedure for detection of meningeal tumor in asymptomatic patients is limited, as demonstrated by Nugent and colleagues (57). They found that cytological evaluation was negative in 56 consecutive patients subjected to lumbar puncture at the time of diagnosis. In the detection of carcinomatous meningitis, it should be emphasized that repeated lumbar punctures are often necessary to detect malignant cells.

Widespread dissemination from small-cell carcinoma also includes metastases to organs such as the pancreas, adrenals and the abdominal lymph nodes, as observed at autopsy. The value of diagnostic procedures such as tumor-seeking isotopes, gallium and whole-body CT scan still remains uncertain. The methods are characterized by being unspecific, unless simultaneous needle biopsy is performed. Metastases to the above-mentioned organs are often clinically silent and do not present special therapeutic problems. Hence, detection of metastases at these locations plays a minor role. Furthermore, metastases to these organs are usually accompanied by metastases to the liver, bone marrow and brain.

Therapy

The treatment of patients with small-cell lung cancer continues to undergo changes and refinement. The 1970's brought considerable progress with a 4—5-fold prolongation of the median survival, including the observation that 5—8% of all patients will achieve long-term remission of several years duration, if not cure. Further therapeutic improvements have not yet been observed in the early 1980's, but the majority of studies published within the last couple of years has consolidated the results from the last decade.

Combination chemotherapy including active agents such as vincristine, cyclophosphamide, VP-16-213, adriamycin, CCNU and methotrexate continues to be the main mode of treatment. It is also well established, based on a number of controlled trials, that the combined use of chemotherapy and radiotherapy is superior to radiotherapy alone. The most recent study focusing on the latter point has been performed by the South-Eastern Cancer Study Group in the U.S.A., who evaluated chemotherapy compared to no chemotherapy in patients staged as having limited disease, with all patients receiving radiotherapy to both chest and brain (42, 60). Patients who received chemotherapy consisting of cyclophosphamide, adriamycin and dimethyl-triazeno-imidazole-carboxamide (DTIC) at the onset of the disease had a significantly longer duration of response than those who were treated initially with radiation therapy alone. No significant difference was shown in the median survival, which might be explained by the fact that patients who received radiotherapy alone at the time of progression all later received chemotherapy.

The question whether combination chemotherapy is superior to single-agent chemotherapy has also been positively answered recently in a study by the Cancer and Acute Leukemia Group B (49). In this trial, 258 patients were randomized to 4 different treatments. In addition, the investigation is shedding light on the question of maintenance therapy. The study design indicated that if patients achieved a complete response after 6 courses of chemotherapy, the patients were randomized to receive maintenance therapy using the induction regime every other month or no maintenance therapy at all. Thirty-six patients with limited disease achieved a complete remission. The remission duration was not significantly prolonged, being 4.0 months for maintenance versus 3.7 months for no maintenance therapy. However, the group who received maintenance therapy lived significantly longer compared to the non-maintained group (16.8 months versus 6.8 months) ($P = 0.01$). Only 11 patients with extensive disease achieved a complete remission: the number of patients in this group randomized to the maintenance phase was too small to allow any conclusions.

At present, it is uncertain what the optimal length of treatment should be, when combination chemotherapy is used. The majority of clinical trials are at present maintaining chemotherapy at periods varying from 6 to 24 months.

With regard to combination chemotherapy, the results of a number of Phase II trials in 1980 and 1981 using intensive combination chemotherapy, with or without radiotherapy, are shown in Tables 3 and 4.

A response is usually obtained in 80–90% of all patients, with a complete response in 15–25%. The median survival for patients with limited disease is approximately 14–16 months, whereas patients with extensive disease obtain a median survival of 8–11 months.

An encouraging sign in the overall management of patients with small-cell carcinoma is the presence of the first reports on the presence of patients with long-term survival. Matthews and colleagues have reported on 121 patients collected from various countries living for more than 2 years after initiation of treatment (48). The diagnosis of small-cell anaplastic carcinoma, including subtyping according to the WHO classification, was verified by a panel of experienced lung pathologists. The patients had undergone various forms of therapy, such as surgery, radiotherapy and chemotherapy – often combined. In analysing the data, Matthews and colleagues conclude that:

1. Special histological subtypes do not appear to account for long-term survival.

Treatment	No. of patients	No. of responders			Response rate (%)	Median duration of response (mth)	Median survival (mth)	Reference
		CR	PR	Total				
Adriamycin Methotrexate Vincristine	19	–	–	4	21	–	–	24
Cyclophosphamide Adriamycin Vincristine alternating with BCNU Methotrexate Procarbazine	31	5	17	22	71	7 (range 1–25 +)	11.5 LD 7.5 ED	65
Adriamycin Vincristine Methotrexate Cyclophosphamide	24	–	–	14	59	–	–	68
CCNU Adriamycin	18	5	5	10	55	4.9	6.5	73
CCNU Adriamycin Procarbazine Vincristine	22	2	7	9	41	3.5	7.7	73
Cyclophosphamide Adriamycin VP-16-213	54	14	28	42	78	13 CR 8 PR	:5 LD 9.5 ED	1

LD = limited disease; ED = extensive disease; CR = complete response; PR = partial response.

TABLE 4. *Combined chemotherapy + radiotherapy in small-cell anaplastic carcinoma, Phase II trials*

Chemotherapy	Radiotherapy Chest	Radiotherapy Brain	No. of patients	Response rate (%) CR	PR	Total	Median duration of response (mth)	Median survival (mth)	Comments	Reference
Cyclophosphamide Vincristine Methotrexate	+	(+)	28	61	21	82	–	9	Prophylactic brain irradiation only given to 18 of 28 patients	69
Cyclophosphamide Vincristine Procarbazine Methotrexate + CF	+	–	56	–	–	55	–	8	Response rate assessed after chemotherapy alone	25
Adriamycin Cyclophosphamide Vincristine	+		26 LD 24 ED	76 50	– –	– –	9.5 5	21 10	Including only patients with Karnofsky >70	63, 64
Cyclophosphamide Adriamycin Vincristine Methotrexate	+		7 LD 28 ED	43 18	29 57	72 75	– –	– 7½	Excessive toxicity	46
Cyclophosphamide Vincristine CCNU Procarbazine	+	–	26	77	16	93	–	10.7	–	11

TABLE 4. *Combined chemotherapy + radiotherapy in small-cell anaplastic carcinoma, Phase II trials (continued)*

Chemotherapy	Radiotherapy		No. of patients	Response rate (%)			Median duration of response (mth)	Median survival (mth)	Comments	Reference
	Chest	Brain		CR	PR	Total				
Adriamycin Cyclophosphamide Vincristine	+	+	33 LD 17 ED	67 12	18 59	85 71		11 + 8	Methotrexate CCNU, and VP-16 used as maintenance therapy	53
Adriamycin Cyclophosphamide Vincristine followed by Procarbazine CCNU Methotrexate	+	–	61 LD 90 ED	24 –	– –	83} 53}	4	11 3	CR increased to 58% after radio-therapy	23

CF = citrovorum factor; CR = complete response; PR = partial response; LD = limited disease; ED = excessive disease.

2. Stage is obviously an important prognostic factor; however, some patients with widespread metastases also achieve long-term, disease-free survival.
3. Survival >5 years offers some hope of freedom from disease. Relapses are seldom recorded beyond 5 years after discontinuation of therapy.

Similar conclusions have been drawn by the Finsen group in Copenhagen, based on a detailed analysis of 4 randomized trials, performed in the period 1973–1977 and including 337 consecutive patients with small-cell carcinoma (29). All patients were carefully staged initially and restaged after 18 months of intensive chemotherapy. In contrast to the previous report, the latter permits an evaluation of the overall results achieved in an unselected group of patients. 15% of all patients were alive after 18 months, including 9% in clinically complete remission, consisting of 7% initially with limited disease and 2% with extensive disease, including liver and bone metastases. Long-term survivors included both patients who had received combined chemo- and radiotherapy and patients who had received chemotherapy alone. A follow-up of this group of patients has indicated that 70% of all patients free from disease at 18 months continue to be disease-free, with the longest follow-up at present being 7 years.

From Switzerland, similar experience has been reported recently (39). Most of the Swiss patients who achieved a long-term remission of more than 2 years presented with localized disease. The report also includes a few patients who initially presented with histologically verified metastases to bone marrow and liver.

Another key question in many current clinical trials is the use of alternating combination chemotherapy. Several groups have attempted to prevent drug resistance to therapy by the early introduction of a second non-cross-resistant drug combination after an initial response to the first combination. Several of the studies are ongoing or have just been completed, but not published. Based on preliminary results, there is evidence of a slight improvement in response duration with the use of alternating drug combinations, but the impact on survival appears to be modest (19, 43, 70). Further detailed analyses of these studies are necessary before definite conclusions can be drawn.

The scheduling of drug administration has been the topic of other clinical trials. Flow-cytometric examinations have demonstrated sequential changes in the tumor cell-cycle distributions following chemotherapy (72). Drug combinations are now being designed to take advantage of the cell-cycle changes induced by the initial therapy. Whether these approaches will improve the therapeutic results has still to be seen. In any case, these studies may increase our understanding of how to schedule the drugs.

Other options for improving systemic therapy are the development of new agents with high activity in small-cell anaplastic carcinoma, particularly drugs which are effective in patients resistant to present therapy. Table 5 shows the results of the many Phase II trials performed within the last few years. Of the many compounds tested in small-cell carcinoma, vindesine and cisplatin appear to have some activity in patients previously treated. It is noteworthy that vindesine is also active in patients who have previously received vincristine. The results with cisplatin are somewhat conflicting, with reported response rates varying from 6 to 31%. It is of interest that Eagan and colleagues found that the addition of low doses of cisplatin to an active treatment program of 3 other cytostatic agents, consisting of cyclophosphamide, VP-16-213 and adriamycin, did not affect the response rate or survival in newly diagnosed patients with small-cell carcinoma (21, 22). Thus, it is possible that the different response rates obtained with cisplatin may be related to the dosage.

Radiotherapy

Small-cell carcinoma of the lung is known to be the most radiosensitive of all lung cancers, but the place of radiotherapy in its management still remains to be defined. At present, radiotherapy is mainly used either as prophylactic brain irradiation in an attempt to reduce the incidence of CNS metastases or in the management of patients presenting with intrathoracic disease alone.

Prophylactic irradiation has been used because CNS metastases have been recognized as a frequent complication of small-cell anaplastic carcinoma. CNS involvement occurs in 50% of all cases (based on autopsy data), probably with an increasing incidence after better systemic treatment has been developed. Major randomized studies on the use of prophylactic irradiation have recently been published (28, 49). None of the studies observed a significant difference in median survival, comparing patients receiving brain irradiation versus no irradiation. The study by the CALGB group demonstrated, however, a significant difference in CNS relapse with only 3 of 79 (4%) relapsing in the brain, after having received prophylactic CNS irradiation, while 15 out of 84 (18%) of the control patients relapsed at this site (P = 0.09) (49). The time to brain relapse was significantly longer in those receiving prophylactic irradiation. If one looks only at the responding patients, there continues to be a highly significant difference in the percentage of relapses in the brain (8/42) for the control patients compared to 3.9% (2/51) for the CNS-irradiated patients (P = 0.02). The discrepancy between the CALGB study and the Copenhagen study (28), which did not reveal any dif-

TABLE 5. *Phase II trials with single agents in small-cell carcinoma of the lung, 1980–1981*

Drug	Dosage and schedule	No. of patients			No. of responders	Response rate (%)	Median duration of response (wk)	Reference
		PT	NT	Total				
Prednimustine	130–220 mg/m² daily for 5 days q. 3 weeks	19	9	28	3	11	8	37
BCNU + amphotericin B	250 mg/m² i.v. q. 8 weeks	–	–	3	1	33	4	61
Vindesine	4 mg/m² i.v. weekly	32	–	32	7	27	7	76
Vindesine	3 mg/m² i.v.	24	–	24	5	21	8	52
5-Fluorouracil	400–600 mg/m² i.v. daily × 5 q. 3 weeks	24	–	24	3	12	6	31
Cisplatin	80 mg/m² i.v. q. 3 weeks	22	1	23	5	22	13	12
Cisplatin	100 mg/m² i.v. q. 3 weeks	18	–	18	1	6	5	44
Cisplatin	120 mg/m² i.v. q. 3 weeks	10	3	13	4	31	14	18

TABLE 5. *Phase II trials with single agents in small-cell carcinoma of the lung, 1980–1981 (continued)*

Drug	Dosage and schedule	No. of patients			No. of responders	Response rate (%)	Median duration of response (wk)	Reference
		PT	NT	Total				
AMSA	35 mg/m² daily × 3 q. 4 weeks	8	0	8	0	0	0	55
AMSA	90–120 mg/m² i.v. q. 3 weeks	13	0	13	0	0	0	15
Triazinate	250 mg/m² i.v. daily × 3 q. 3–4 weeks	0	5	5	2	40	40	13
Procarbazine	100–120 mg/m² p.o. daily × 14 q. 4 weeks	24	0	24	0	0	—	59

PT = previously treated with chemotherapy/radiotherapy; NT = not treated.

45

ference, may be due to the time at which the prophylactic brain irradiation was given. In the CALGB study, it was given at the onset of therapy, while CNS irradiation was applied 12 weeks after the initiation of therapy in the other study. Another explanation may be that CCNU was included as part of the combination chemotherapy in the Finsen study, and not in the study by the CALGB. However, the study by the South-Eastern Cooperative Group (42) and some of the non-randomized trials using prophylactic brain irradiation also indicate that the frequency of occurrence can be reduced by prophylactic brain irradiation (20). The lack of influence of prophylactic brain irradiation on survival is probably due to inability to control the disease outside the CNS system. With regard to the dose of radiotherapy, most investigators are applying doses ranging from 3000 rads in 2 weeks to 4000 rads in 3 weeks, given no later than 12 weeks after initiation of chemotherapy. At present, it appears that prophylactic brain irradiation, if used, should be limited to patients achieving complete remission, because patients achieving only a partial response remain at a high risk for further spread of the tumor to the CNS system. It is conceivable that prophylactic CNS irradiation will become more important in the future, if there is further improvement in systemic treatment.

Meningeal metastases likewise appear to be a more common finding in connection with the overall improvement of survival. In autopsy studies, meningeal metastases were found in 12% of patients. The occurrence of meningeal carcinomatoses is generally associated with extensive disease and systemic relapse (2, 4). However, meningeal metastases have also been reported to be the only evidence of disease, both at relapse and at autopsy. The treatment of meningeal metastases includes intraspinal administration of chemotherapy, with or without irradiation of the spine and brain. Independent of intensive therapy, survival is usually no more than 2–3 months after the diagnosis of meningeal carcinomatosis has been made.

The role of radiotherapy of the primary tumor and regional lymph nodes in the overall management of small-cell carcinoma still remains to be clarified. Several studies have addressed this question, using various types of combination chemotherapy and radiotherapy in various schedules and dosages, but detailed information and thus conclusive data are still lacking from these studies. At present, the trend in the randomized trials indicates that the use of local radiotherapy to the primary tumor does decrease the incidence and delay the time of local recurrence, while the complete response rates and median survival are not influenced. Whether the use of a combined modality of treatment using combination chemotherapy and radiotherapy will result in an increase in long-term survival, remains to be seen.

The optimal way to combine the two modalities is also under investigation, and many trials are particularly focusing on ways to reduce the considerable toxicity of the combined treatments, including esophagitis, pneumonitis and myelotoxicity. The schedule and dosage of radiotherapy to be used to obtain long-term local control of the disease remain uncertain. It is expected that the increased use of CT scanning will result in the reduction of treatment volumes, thereby minimizing radiation damage to normal lung tissue and to the esophagus.

Other modalities of treatment

With the lack of significant progress in the last 2–3 years, it is not surprising that various other therapy modalities are being tested. Noteworthy is the exploration of total body irradiation and the introduction of autologous bone marrow transplantation, combined with high-dose chemotherapy. In the study by Qasim and The (62), 17 patients with small-cell anaplastic carcinoma underwent total body irradiation. Eight patients had documented distant metastases at the onset of therapy. The treatment consisted of total body irradiation as 100 rads mid-plain 5 times a week for the first 2 weeks. In the 3rd week, irradiation to the primary tumor, the whole mediastinum and both supraclavicular foci was given with a total dose of 4000 rads mid-plain in 20 fractions over 4 weeks. In the last week of treatment, the irradiation field was extended to include the liver and the dose of 1000 rads mid-plain was given to the liver in 5 fractions in 1 week. The entire treatment was given on an outpatient basis. Among 7 patients with extensive disease, 2 partial remissions of 3.5 months duration were observed, while all patients with localized disease were responding. Of the 9 patients however, 5 have relapsed. The overall median duration of response was 6 months (median 3–9 + months). Another pilot study of total body irradiation was performed by Byhardt and colleagues (7). In this study, irradiation of the primary tumor was given first; the patients were then randomized to receive either total body irradiation or combination chemotherapy. All 8 patients failed on total body irradiation, as they developed evidence of metastases 2–12 months afterwards. Some of these patients were subsequently put on chemotherapy with good response.

Data on bone marrow transplantation have been published by Spitzer and colleagues (67). Nineteen patients with solid tumors including 9 patients with small-cell carcinoma, who all had earlier received extensive chemotherapy, received high-dose chemotherapy followed by autologous bone marrow infusion. The chemotherapy consisted of cyclophosphamide (2–6 g/m^2 i.v.), VP-16 (500–600 mg/m^2 i.v.) and CCNU

(300 mg/m^2 p.o.). One complete response and 4 partial responses were observed in 6 patients with evaluable disease and, of these, 1 patient achieved a complete remission of 12 weeks duration, while there were 4 partial remissions varying from 7 to 55 + weeks. Further studies along these lines are awaited with interest.

Another modality has been the use of anticoagulants in the overall treatment of small-cell carcinoma. In an interesting study by the VA Lung Study Group, patients were randomized to receive combination chemotherapy and radiotherapy, with or without warfarin (75). A total of 50 patients was included in the study, with 25 patients in each group. Chemotherapy included cyclophosphamide, vincristine and methotrexate; radiotherapy consisted of 3200 rads to the primary tumor and primary draining area in the mediastinum. Warfarin was administered to patients in doses intended to prolong the prothrombin time to approximately twice the control value. The median survival for 25 control patients was 24 weeks and for 25 warfarin-treated patients 50 weeks ($P = 0.026$). The difference between the two groups could not be accounted for by differences in performance status, stage of disease, age or sex. The survival advantage associated with warfarin administration was observed both for patients with extensive disease and for those who failed to achieve a complete or partial remission. The warfarin-treated group also demonstrated a significant increase in time to first evidence of disease progression. The study suggests, therefore, that warfarin may be useful in the treatment of small-cell carcinoma. Further studies should proceed along these lines.

Conclusions

Summarizing the data from the literature in 1980–1981, the following conclusions concerning the treatment of small-cell carcinoma can be reached:
1. Combination chemotherapy including agents such as vincristine, adriamycin, cyclophosphamide, VP-16, CCNU and methotrexate continues to be the main mode of treatment of the disease. An objective response can be achieved within 1–2 months after the initiation of therapy in 80–90% of all patients, including a complete response in 20–25%. The duration of remission will usually last 9–12 months, resulting in an overall survival for patients with localized disease of 14–16 months and for patients with extensive disease of 8–11 months. 5–10% of all patients will achieve long-term remissions, lasting from 2 to 7 + years.
2. Combined use of chemotherapy and radiotherapy is clearly superior to radiotherapy alone.

3. Prophylactic brain irradiation decreases the incidence of brain metastases, but it does not change the overall median survival. It should probably be restricted to patients who have achieved complete remission.
4. Radiotherapy to the primary tumor and including the regional lymph nodes decreases the rate of local recurrence, but it does not influence the median survival when given with combination chemotherapy. The morbidity of the combined modality of therapy is considerably higher than when using chemotherapy alone. Whether the percentage of long-term remission survivors is higher when the combined modality of therapy is used, is still uncertain.
5. With regard to maintenance treatment with combination chemotherapy, at least one randomized trial has shown that therapy continued for 2 years is superior to treatment for 6 months alone.
6. A number of ongoing studies are exploring the use of cyclic non-cross-resistant combination chemotherapy to increase the complete response rate and to prolong the duration of remission.
7. Among new compounds, vindesine and cisplatin have shown some activity in small-cell anaplastic carcinoma.
8. The first reports have emerged describing the features of long-term survivors, including patients who initially presented with advanced disease.
9. Basic research in the last two years has provided substantial new information on the biology of small-cell carcinoma. It is expected that this information will lead to more rational treatment programs in the years to come.

References

1. Abeloff, M.D., Ettinger, D.S., Order, S.E., Khouri, N., Mellits, E.D., Dorschel, N.T. and Baumgardner, R. (1981): Intensive introduction chemotherapy in 54 patients with small cell carcinoma of the lung. *Cancer Treat. Rep., 65,* 639–646.
2. Aisner, J., Ostrow, S., Govindan, S. and Wiernik, P.H. (1981): Leptomeningeal carcinomatosis in small cell carcinoma of the lung. *Med. pediat. Oncol., 9,* 47–59.
3. Alvarez, R., Gazdar, A.F., Carney, D.N., Dermody, W.C., Bunn, P.A. and Minna, J.D. (1981): Clonal heterogeneity of small cell carcinoma of the lung (SCCL). *Proc. Amer. Soc. clin. Oncol.,* 339.
4. Aroney, R.S., Dalley, D.N., Chan, W.K., Bell, D.R. and Levi, J.A. (1981): Meningeal carcinomatosis in small cell carcinoma of the lung. *Amer. J. Med., 71,* 26–32.
5. Baylin, S.B. and Gazdar, A.F. (1981): Endocrine biochemistry in the spectrum of human lung cancer: implications for the cellular origin of small cell

carcinoma. In: *Small Cell Lung Cancer 1981*, pp. 123–145. Editors: F.A. Greco, R.K. Oldham and P.A. Bunn. Grune and Stratton, New York.

6. Bergevin, P.R. (1980): Small-cell bronchogenic carcinoma *N.Y. J. Med., 80,* 1847–1850.
7. Byhardt, R.W., Cox, J.D., Wilson, J.F., Libnoch, J. and Stein, R.S. (1979): Total body irradiation vs. chemotherapy as a systemic adjuvant for small cell carcinoma of the lung. *Int. J. Radiat. Oncol. biol. Phys., 5,* 2043–2048.
8. Burdon, J.G., Sinclair, R.A. and Henderson, M.M. (1979): Small cell carcinoma of the lung: prognosis in relation to histologic subtypes. *Chest, 76,* 302–304.
9. Carney, D.N., Bunn, P.A., Gazdar, A.F., Pagan, J.A. and Minna, J.D. (1981): Selective growth in serum-free hormone-supplemented medium of tumor cells obtained by biopsy from patients with small cell carcinoma of the lung. *Proc. nat. Acad. Sci. U.S.A., 78,* 3185–3189.
10. Carney, D.N., Matthews, M.J., Ihde, D.C., Bunn, P.A., Cohen, M.H., Makuch, R.W., Gazdar A.F. and Minna, J.D. (1981): Influence of histologic subtype of small cell carcinoma of the lung or clinical presentation, response to therapy and survival. *J. nat. Cancer Inst., 65,* 1225–1229.
11. Carrière, J.C., Léophonte, P., Armand, J.P., Daly, N., Pons, A., Carles, P. and Carton, M. (1979): Cancer pulmonaire à petites cellules: traitement par association chimiothérapie (COPP-CCNU) et radiothérapie. *Rev. Méd. Toulouse, 15,* 75–79.
12. Cavalli, F., Jungi, W.F. and Sonntag, R.W. (1979): Phase II trial of cis-dichlorodiamineplatinum (II) in advanced malignant lymphoma and small cell lung cancer: preliminary results. *Cancer Treat. Rep., 63,* 1599–1603.
13. Creagan, E.T., Eagan, R.T., Fleming, T.R., Frytak, S., Ingle, J.N., Kvols, L.K. and Nichols, W.C. (1980): Phase II evaluation of triazinate in patients with metastatic lung cancer. *Cancer Treat. Rep., 64,* 1057–1059.
14. Cuttitta, F., Rosen, S., Abrams, P., Gazdar, F., Schwade, J. and Minna, J. (1981): Monoclonal antibodies (MAs) which react with several types of human lung cancer. *Proc. Amer. Soc. clin. Oncol.,* 374.
15. Dady, P.J., Sappino, A.-P., Rudd, A. and Smith, I.E. (1981): A phase II clinical study of m-AMSA in small cell carcinoma of the lung. *Cancer Chemother. Pharmacol., 6,* 195–196.
16. Davis, S. and Sobel, H. (1981): Histologic subtypes of small cell carcinoma of the lung: response to therapy. *Eur. J. Cancer, 17,* 351–354.
17. Davis, S., Stanley, K.E., Yesner, R., Kuang, D.T. and Morris, J.F. (1981): Small cell carcinoma of the lung - survival according to histologic subtype. *Cancer, 47,* 1863–1866.
18. De Jager, R., Longeval, E. and Klastersky, J. (1981): High-dose cisplatin with fluid and mannitol-induced diuresis in advanced lung cancer: a phase II clinical trial of the EORTC Lung Cancer Working Party (Belgium). *Cancer Treat. Rep., 64,* 1341–1346.
19. Dombernowsky, P., Hansen, H.H., Sörenson, S. and Österlind, K. (1979): Sequential versus non-sequential combination chemotherapy using 6 drugs in advanced small cell carcinoma (sm.a.c.): a comparative trial including 146 patients. *Proc. Amer. Ass. Cancer Res., 20,* 277.

20. Eagan, R., Frytag, S., Lee, R.E., Eagan, E.T., Ingle, J.N. and Nichols, W.C. (1981): A case for preplanned thoracic and prophylactic whole brain irradiation therapy in limited small-cell lung cancer. *Cancer clin. Trials, 4,* 261–266.

21. Eagan, R.T., Frytak, S., Nichols, W.C., Ingle, J.N., Creagan, E.T. and Kvols, L.K. (1981): Cyclophosphamide and VP-16-213 with or without cisplatin in squamous cell and small cell lung cancers. *Cancer Treat. Rep., 65,* 453–458.

22. Eagan, R.T., Lee, R.E., Frytak, S., Fleming, T.R., Ingle, J.N., Creagan, E.T., Nichols, W.C., Kvols, L.K. and Coles, D.T. (1981): An evaluation of low-dose cis-platin as part of combined modality therapy of limited small cell lung cancer. *Cancer clin. Trials, 4,* 267–271.

23. Feld, R., Pringle, J., Evans, W.K., Keen, C.W., Quirt, J.C., Curtis, J.E., Baker, M.S., Yeoh, J.L., Deboer, G. and Brown, T.C. (1981): Combined modality treatment of small cell carcinoma of the lung. *Arch. intern. Med., 141,* 469–473.

24. Fréour, P., Chauvergne, J., Courty, G., Taytard, A., Bordas, J., Hoerni, B., Chomy, P. and Roquain, J. (1980): Polychimiothérapie des cancers bronchiques inopérables par une association d'adriamycine, vincristine et méthotrexate. *Bordeaux méd., 13,* 185–190.

25. Gregor, A., Morgan, P.G.M., Morgen, R.L., Scadding, F.H. and Turner-Warwick, M. (1977): Small cell carcinoma: combined approach to treatment. *Thorax, 34,* 789–793.

26. Hansen, H.H., Dombernowsky, P., Hansen, M. and Hirsch, F. (1978): Chemotherapy of advanced small-cell anaplastic carcinoma: superiority in a randomized trial of a 4-drug combination to a 3-drug combination. *Ann. intern. Med., 89,* 177–181.

27. Hansen, H.H. (1980): Management of small cell anaplastic carcinoma. In: *Lung Cancer 1980,* pp. 113–133. Editors: H.H. Hansen and M. Rørth. Excerpta Medica, Amsterdam–Oxford.

28. Hansen, H.H., Dombernowsky, P., Hirsch, F.R., Hansen, M. and Rygård, J. (1980): Prophylactic irradiation in bronchogenic small cell anaplastic carcinoma. *Cancer, 46,* 279–284.

29. Hansen, M., Hansen, H.H. and Dombernowsky, P. (1980): Long-term survival in small cell carcinoma of the lung. *J. Amer. med. Ass., 244,* 247–250.

30. Harper, P.G., Houang, M., Spiro, S.G., Geddes, D., Hodson, M. and Souhami, R.L. (1981): Computerized axial tomography in the pretreatment assessment of small-cell carcinoma of the bronchus. *Cancer, 47,* 1775–1780.

31. Havsteen, H., Sörenson, S., Rørth, M., Dombernowsky, P. and Hansen, H.H. (1981): 5-Fluorouracil in the treatment of advanced small-cell anaplastic carcinoma of the lung: a phase II trial. *Cancer Treat. Rep., 65,* 123–125.

32. Hirsch, F.R., Paulson, O., Vraa-Jensen, J. and Hansen, H.H. (1981): Intracranial metastases in small cell carcinoma of the lung: correlation of clinical and autopsy findings. *Cancer,* in press.

33. Hirsch, F.R., Matthews, M.J. and Yesner, R. (1982): Histopathologic

classification of small cell carcinoma of the lung: comments based on an interobserver examination. *Cancer,* in press.

34. Hirsch, R.F., Østerlind, K. and Hansen, H.H. (1982): The prognostic implications of histopathologic subtyping of small cell carcinoma of the lung. *Cancer,* submitted for publication.

35. Ihde, D.C., Dunnich, N.R., Johnston-Early, A., Bunn, P.A., Cohen, M.H. and Minna, J.D. (1980): Abdominal computed tomography in small cell lung cancer: assessment of extent of disease and response to treatment. In: *Abstracts, II World Conference on Lung Cancer, 1980,* p. 55. Editors: H.H. Hansen and P. Dombernowsky. Excerpta Medica, Amsterdam−Oxford−Princeton.

36. Ikegami, H., Horai, T. and Hattori, S. (1981): Combined modality studies on small cell carcinoma of the lung: current status in Japan. In: *New Drugs in Cancer Chemotherapy,* pp. 257−266. Editors: S.K. Carter, Y. Sakurai and H. Umezawa. Springer-Verlag, Berlin.

37. Jensen, S.H., Hansen, H.H. and Dombernowsky, P. (1980): Phase II trial of prednimustine (NSC-134087) in the treatment of small-cell anaplastic carcinoma of the lung. *Cancer Chemother. Pharmacol., 4,* 259−261.

38. Joss, R., Goldhirsch, A. and Brunner, K.W. (1980): Das anaplastische kleinzellige Bronchuskarzinom. *Dtsch. med. Wschr., 105,* 732−735.

39. Joss, R., Kapanci, Y., Widmann, J.J., Brunner, K.W. and Alberto, P. (1981): Langfristig tumorfrei überlebende Patienten mit anaplastischem kleinzelligen Bronchuskarzinom. *Schweiz. med. Wschr., 111,* 1282−1286.

40. Knost, J. and Greco, F.A. (1980): Limited stage small cell lung cancer. *J. Tenn. med. Ass., 73,* 578−582.

41. Klastersky, J. (1980): Kleinzelliges Bronchuskarzinom: Aussichten auf eine kurative Behandlung. *Ars Med., 5,* 238−241.

42. Krauss, S., Perez, C., Lowenbraun, S., Sonoda, T., Bartolucci, A. and Buchanan, R. (1980): Combined modality treatment of localized small-cell lung carcinoma. *Cancer clin. Trials, 3,* 297−306.

43. Krauss, S., Lowenbraun, S., Bartolucci, R. and Birch, R. (1981): Alternatively non-cross-resistant drug combination in the treatment of metastatic small-cell carcinoma of the lung. *Cancer clin. Trials, 4,* 147−153.

44. Levenson, R.M., Ihde Jr., D.C., Hubermann, M.S., Cohen, M.H., Bunn, P.A. and Minna, J.D. (1981): Phase II trial of cis-platin in small cell carcinoma of the lung. *Cancer Treat. Rep., 65,* 905−907.

45. Livingston, R.B. (1980): Small cell carcinoma of the lung. *Blood, 56,* 575−584.

46. Livingston, R.B., Mira, J., Haas, C. and Heilbrun, L. (1979): Unexpected toxicity of combined modality therapy for small cell carcinoma of the lung. *Int. J. Radiat. Oncol. biol. Phys., 5,* 1637−1641.

47. Matthews, M.J. and Gazdar, A.F. (1981): Pathology of small cell carcinoma of the lung and its subtypes: a clinico-pathologic correlation. In: *Lung Cancer,* pp. 283−306. Editor: R.B. Livingston. Martinus Nijhoff Publishers, The Hague.

48. Matthews, M.J., Rozencweig, M., Staquet, M.J., Minna, J.D. and Muggia, F.M. (1979): Long-term survivors with small cell carcinoma of the lung. *Eur. J. Cancer, 16,* 527−531.

49. Maurer, L.H., Tulloh, M., Weiss, R.B., Blom, J., Leone, L., Glidewell, O. and Pajak, T.F. (1980): A randomized combined modality trial in small cell carcinoma of the lung. *Cancer, 45,* 30–39.
50. Mercke, C. and Lagercrantz, R. (1980): Framsteg i behandlingen av småcellig bronkialcancer. *Läkartidningen, 77,* 1919–1921.
51. Meyer, J.A. and Parker, F.B. (1980): Small cell carcinoma of the lung. *Ann. thorac. Surg., 30,* 602–610.
52. Natale, R.B., Gralia, R.J. and Wittes, R.E. (1981): Phase II trial of vindesine in patients with small cell lung carcinoma. *Cancer Treat Rep, 65,* 129–131.
53. Niederle, N., Seeber, S., Konietzko, N. and Schmidt, C.G. (1980): Kombinierte Chemo- und Radiotherapie (ACO II plus RT) des inoperablen kleinzelligen und anaplastisch-grosszelligen Bronchialkarzinoms. *Prax. Pneumol., 34,* 533–540.
54. Niewig, O.E., Beekhuis, H., Piers, D.A., Woldring, M.S., Van der Wal, A.M. and Sluiks, H.J. (1980): Detection and staging of lung cancer with [57]Co-bleomycin and ^{67}Ga-citrate scintigraphy. In: *Abstracts, II World Conference on Lung Cancer, 1980,* p. 59. Editors: H.H. Hansen and P. Dombernowsky. Excerpta Medica, Amsterdam–Oxford–Princeton.
55. Nichols, W.C., Eagan, R.T., Frytak, S., Ingle, J.N., Creagan, E.T. and Kvols, L.K. (1980): Phase II evaluation of AMSA in patients with metastatic lung cancer. *Cancer Treat. Rep., 64,* 1383–1385.
56. North, W.G., Maurer, L.H., Valtin, H. and O'Donnell, J.F. (1980): Human neurophysins as potential tumor markers for small cell carcinoma of the lung: application of specific radioimmunoassays. *J. clin. Endocr., 51,* 892–896.
57. Nugent, J.L., Bunn, P.A., Matthews, M.J., Ihde, D.C., Cohen, M.H., Gazdar, A. and Minna, J.D. (1979): CNS metastases in small cell bronchogenic carcinoma: increasing frequency and changing pattern with lengthening survival. *Cancer, 44,* 1885–1893.
58. Oldham, R.K. and Greco, F.A. (1980): Small-cell lung cancer: a curable disease. *Cancer Chemother. Pharmacol., 4,* 173–177.
59. Pedersen, A.G., Sörenson, S., Aabo, K., Dombernowsky, P. and Hansen, H.H. (1982): Phase II study of procarbazine in small cell carcinoma of the lung. *Cancer Treat. Rep., 66,* in press.
60. Perez, C.A., Krauss, S., Bartolucci, A.A., Durant, J.R., Lowenbraun, S., Salter, M.M., Storaasli, J., Kellermeyer, R., Comas, F. and The South Eastern Cancer Study Group (1981): Thoracic and elective brain irradiation with concomitant or delayed multiagent chemotherapy in the treatment of localized small cell carcinoma of the lung. *Cancer, 47,* 2407–2413.
61. Presant, C., Hillinger, S. and Klahr, C. (1980): Phase II study of 1,3-bis(2-chloroethyl)-1-nitrosourea (BCNU, NSC-409962) with amphotericin B in bronchogenic carcinoma. *Cancer, 45,* 6–10.
62. Qasim, M.M. and The, S.K. (1979): Combined total body irradiation and local radiation therapy in oat cell carcinoma of the bronchus. *Clin. Radiol., 30,* 161–163.
63. Seeber, S., Niederle, N., Schilcher, R.B. and Schmidt, C.G. (1980): Adriamycin, Cyclophosphamide und Vincristin (ACO) beim kleinzelligen

Bronchialkarzinom: Verlaufsanalyse und Langzeitergebnisse. *Onkologie, 3,* 5–11.

64. Seeber, S., Schilcher, R.B., Swosdyk, P., Sheulen, M.F., Schmidt, C.G., Holfeld, H., Schmitt, G. and Scherer, E. (1980): Kombinierte Chemo- und Radiotherapie bei inoperablem kleinzellig-anaplastischem Bronchialkarzinom. *Dtsch. med. Wschr., 105,* 474–477.

65. Sierocki, J.S., Hilaris, B.S., Hopfan, S., Golbey, R.B. and Wittes, R.E. (1980): Small cell carcinoma of the lung: experience with a six-drug regimen. *Cancer, 45,* 417–422.

66. Sorenson, G.D., Pettengill, O.S. and Cate, C.C. (1981): Studies on xenografts of small cell carcinoma of the lung. In: *Small Cell Lung Cancer,* pp. 95–121. Editors: F.A. Greco, R.K. Oldham and P.A. Bunn. Grune and Stratton, New York.

67. Spitzer, G., Dicke, K.A., Litam, J., Verma, D.S., Zander, A., Lanzotti, V., Valdivieso, M., McCredie, K.B. and Samuels, M.L. (1980): High-dose combination chemotherapy with autologous bone marrow transplantation in adult solid tumors. *Cancer, 45,* 3075–3085.

68. Taytard, A., Chomy, P., Courty, G., Gachie, J.P. and Roquain, J. (1980): Résultats d'une polychimiothérapie séquentielle (adriamycine, vincristine, cyclophosphamide, méthotrexate) dans les carcinomes bronchiques à petites cellules et indifférenciés. *Rev. franç. Mal. resp., 8,* 225–232.

69. Tjho, E.T.T., Keilholz, A. and Broks, P.C. (1980): Resultaten van de behandeling van kleincellig ongedifferentieerd bronchuscarcinoom met de combinatie radio- en chemotherapie. *Ned. T. Geneesk., 15,* 124, 540–544.

70. Vincent, R.G., Wilson, H.E., Lane, W.W., Chen, T.J., Raza, S., Gutierrez, A.C. and Caracandas, J.E. (1981): Progress in chemotherapy of small cell carcinoma of the lung. *Cancer, 47,* 229–235.

71. Vindeløv, L.L., Hansen, H.H., Christensen, I.J., Spang-Thomsen, M. and Hirsch, F.R. (1980): Clonal heterogeneity of small-cell anaplastic carcinoma of the lung demonstrated by flow-cytometric DNA analysis. *Cancer Res., 40,* 4295–4300.

72. Vindeløv, L.L., Hansen, H.H., Gersel, A., Hirsch, F.R. and Nissen, N.I. (1981): Treatment of small cell carcinoma of the lung monitored by sequential flow-cytometric DNA-analysis. *Cancer Res.,* in press.

73. Vogelzang, N.J., Trowbridge, R.C., Frenning, D.H., Theologides, A., Kennedy, B.J., Kelly, D.R., Ewing, S.L. and Vosika, G.J. (1980): Chemotherapy for small cell bronchogenic carcinoma: CCNU and doxorubicin, vincristine and procarbazine. *Cancer Treat. Rep., 64,* 997–1000.

74. Weiss, R.B., Minna, J.D., Glatstein, E., Martini, N., Ihde, D.C. and Muggia, F.M. (1980): Treatment of small cell undifferentiated carcinoma of the lung: update of recent results. *Cancer Treat. Rep., 64,* 539–548.

75. Zacharski, L.R., Henderson, W.G., Rickles, F.R., Forman, W.B., Cornell Jr., C.J., Forcier, R.J., Edwards, R., Headley, E., Kim, S.H., O'Donnell, J.R., O'Dell, R., Tornyos, K. and Kwann, H.C. (1981): Effect of warfarin in small cell carcinoma of the lung. *J. Amer. med. Ass., 245,* 831–835.

76. Østerlind, K., Dombernowsky, P., Sørensen, P.G. and Hansen, H.H. (1981): Vindesine in the treatment of small cell anaplastic carcinoma. *Cancer Treat. Rep.,* in press.

77. Østerlind, K. (1981): Unpublished data.

Hematoporphyrin derivative and photoradiation for tumor localization and treatment of lung cancer*

Yoshihiro Hayata, Harubumi Kato, Chimori Konaka, Motohiko Aida, Jutaro Ono and Katsuaki Nishimiya

To improve the therapeutic results, lung cancer must be detected at an early stage. Much progress has been made in the early detection of peripheral lesions by mass chest X-ray surveys, while sputum cytology surveys of high-risk groups in Japan have proved effective in the detection of central-type lung cancer. Most cases of early-stage, central-type lung cancer can be localized and definitively diagnosed by fiberoptic bronchoscopy. However, some cases, such as those with a negative chest X-ray and positive sputum for occult lung cancer or those with coexisting chronic inflammatory changes in the bronchial wall, can be difficult to localize. While the 5-year survival in resected cases of central-type, early-stage lung cancer is over 90%, showing results comparable to those of breast or stomach cancer, there are some inoperable early-stage cases due to poor pulmonary function or other factors. In the past, chemotherapy or radiation therapy was performed in these cases, but the need for the development of even more effective therapeutic modalities for these cases has been recognized.

Recently, increasing attention has been paid to the possible use of hematoporphyrin derivative (HpD) for localization of early-stage, central-type lung cancer using violet exciting light to elicit fluorescence and for photoradiation therapy (PRT) using red exciting light for cytocidal effects. Based on the results of animal studies, we have been applying these methods clinically in lung cancer and here present our results and discuss their effectiveness.

*Supported in part by a Grant-in-Aid for Scientific Research from the Ministry of Education, a Cancer Research Grant from the Ministry of Welfare, Japan, and a Cancer Research Grant from the Tokyo Medical College Cancer Center.

Material and methods

Hematoporphyrin derivative

HpD, prepared by acetic and sulfuric acid treatment of hematoporphyrin hydrochloride (16), was supplied by Dr. T.J. Dougherty and his associates at Roswell Park Memorial Institute and by Oncology Research and Development Inc. of New York. HpD is known to have a greater affinity for malignant than for normal tissue, it has a 50% clearance in blood of approximately 25 hours for doses of 2.5–5.0 mg/kg body weight (4) and remains for longer periods in malignant than in normal tissue. HpD is excreted through the liver and gastrointestinal tract. The only known side-effect is sensitivity to sunlight (24). HpD emits a red fluorescence with peaks at 630 and 690 nm when excited by violet light with a wavelength of 405 nm. This means that tumors can be localized by observing the red fluorescence emitted by areas of malignancy after a lapse of time following administration to allow HpD to be discharged from normal tissue. Since HpD also produces cytocidal effects in malignant tissue by activation by red light, it has possible therapeutic applications. Red light with a wavelength of 630 nm has good tissue penetration (4, 5). HpD doses of 2.5–5.0 mg/kg body weight were injected intravenously between 48 and 72 hours before diagnostic and therapeutic procedures.

Fluorescence detection (photoradiation)

A krypton ion laser (model 164-11, wavelength 406.7–422.6 nm, 1 W power, Spectra Physics, Mountain View, CA) was used as a source of violet light for excitation of HpD. An interference filter was used to obtain a beam with a wavelength of approximately 406 nm which was transmitted via a 400 μm quartz fiber (Quartz Products, Plainfield, NJ) inserted through the intrumentation channel of a fiberoptic bronchoscope (Olympus 1T) (Fig. 1). An image intensifier, designed by Profio (21), with a 610 nm barrier filter was used to detect fluorescence. The ×30,000 image intensifier is a Varo-8858 and the tube consists of a 3-stage electrostatic focus. Weak red fluorescence is converted to a bright green image.

Therapeutic procedure (photoradiation therapy)

An argon laser (model 171-08, wavelength 457.9–514.5 nm, 15 W power, Spectra Physics) and dye laser (model 375-01, wavelength 630–640 nm) were used with rhodamin B dye to obtain a spectral output of 630 nm. The red light was transmitted via a quartz fiber inserted through the instrumentation channel of the fiberoptic bronchoscope (Fig. 2).

DIAGNOSTIC SYSTEM

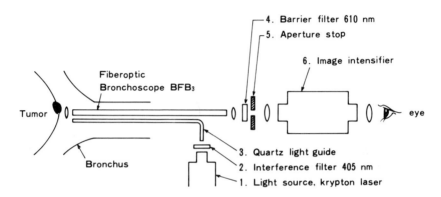

FIG. 1. *Diagram of the krypton ion laser photoradiation system. The laser beam is transmitted via the quartz fiber inserted through the instrumentation channel of the fiberoptic bronchoscope. Fluorescence is observed through an image intensifier.*

THERAPEUTIC SYSTEM

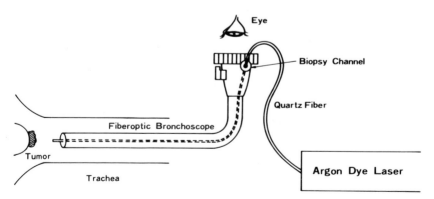

FIG. 2. *Argon dye laser photoradiation system. Red light from the argon dye laser is transmitted via the quartz fiber through the fiberoptic bronchoscope.*

Procedure

For diagnosis, the lesion was irradiated with the krypton ion laser beam, maintaining the tip of the quartz fiber at a distance of 10–30 mm from the focus. For treatment, the tumor was irradiated for 10–30 min at the same distance from the focus with an argon dye laser beam of 100–600 mW power at the fiber tip (Fig. 3).

Experimental study in dogs

Before applying these methods in human cases, we performed photoradiation in 7 experimentally induced canine central-type lung cancer and PRT in 3 dog lung cancers which were induced by weekly submucosal injections of 20-methylcholanthrene at the bifurcation of the right apical and cardiac lobe bronchi. Invasive squamous-cell carcinoma developed as a result of this procedure after a period of 18–26 weeks (8). The results confirmed the safety and effectiveness of photoradiation and PRT (9, 11).

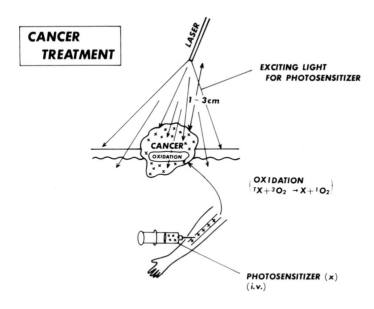

FIG. 3. *Photoradiation procedure. The laser is irradiated from a distance of 10–30 mm with an argon dye laser beam of 100–600 mW power for 10–30 min after i.v. injection of hematoporphyrin derivative.*

Clinical cases

Thirty-five cases of lung cancer, including 3 cases of early-stage central type, and 4 cases of atypical squamous-cell metaplasia were irradiated with krypton ion laser photoradiation to observe fluorescence. PRT was performed in 45 lung cancer cases, including 5 early-stage cases, and in 2 cases of severely atypical squamous-cell metaplasia (Table 1).

Results

Table 2 shows the results of photoradiation in lung cancer cases. Fluorescence was observed in all 3 early-stage cases and in 3 cases of severely atypical squamous-cell metaplasia, but no fluorescence was seen in one case with mildly atypical squamous-cell metaplasia. In Stage I, II, III and IV lung cancer, fluorescence was observed in 29 out of 32 cases. Fluorescence was not seen due to bleeding or necrosis on the tumor surface in 2 cases and because of submucosal growth in another case.

Case 1   Figure 4 is the chest X-ray film of a 60-year-old female who presented with a slight cough. An infiltrative shadow can be seen in the right hilar region. Fiberoptic bronchoscopy revealed only a slight redness at the orifice of the right upper lobe bronchus, but neither tumor nor invasion could be recognized. To differentiate between cancer and bronchitis, photoradiation was performed 48 hours after i.v. injection of HpD 2.5 mg/kg body weight. Slight fluorescence was observed in the anterior portion of the orifice of the right upper lobe

TABLE 1. *Lung cancer cases examined for fluorescence or treated with photoradiation, after administration of hematoporphyrin derivative*

Clinical stage	No. of cases	Fluorescence	Treatment
Early	5	3	5
Stage I	5	4	5
Stage II	9	7	9
Stage III, IV	28	21	26
Total	47	35	45
Atypical squamous metaplasia			
Severe	3	3	2
Mild	1	1	0

Sept. 30, 1981.

TABLE 2. *Results of hematoporphyrin derivative and photoradiation using a krypton ion laser beam*

Clinical stage	No. of cases	Fluorescence	
		Positive	Negative
Lung cancer			
Early stage	3	3	0
Other stages	32	29	3
Total	35	32	3
Atypical squamous metaplasia			
Severe	3	3	0
Mild	1	0	1
Total	4	3	1

Sept. 30, 1981.

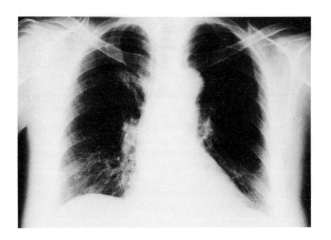

FIG. 4. *Chest X-ray of a 60-year-old female. An infiltrative shadow can be seen in the right hilar region.*

bronchus. Brushing cytology and biopsy were performed at the site of the fluorescent lesion. Cells suggestive of squamous-cell carcinoma were seen in the punch biopsy specimen, but features of severely atypical squamous-cell metaplasia were observed in the brushing cytology specimen.

Case 2   A 74-year-old male presented with cough, but his chest X-ray was negative. Well-differentiated squamous-cell carcinoma cells were observed in his sputum in February, 1981, but there were no abnormal findings on his chest X-ray film. Fiberoptic bronchoscopy revealed two smoothly surfaced tumors, both 2.0 mm in diameter, in right B_2b. The biopsied specimen showed features of squamous-cell carcinoma and photoradiation was performed 48 hours after i.v. injection of HpD 2.5 mg/kg body weight. Fluorescence was observed at the site of the tumors (Fig. 5). PRT was performed in this case after photoradiation and the results are presented below.

Case 3   An infiltrative shadow was detected in the left upper lung field in the chest X-ray of a 50-year-old male complaining of bloody sputum and cough. Fiberoptic bronchoscopy revealed an irregular tumor in the left upper lobe bronchus. Biopsy of the lesion showed features of poorly differentiated adenocarcinoma. Photoradiation was performed 72 hours after i.v. injection of HpD 2.5 mg/kg body weight and fluorescence was observed at the site of tumor invasion (Fig. 6).

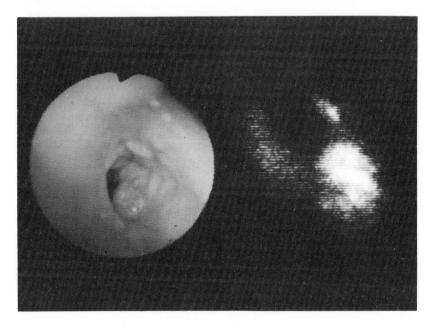

FIG. 5.   *Photoradiation in a 74-year-old male with squamous-cell carcinoma. Two smoothly surfaced tumors 2.0 mm in diameter can be seen in right B_2b (left). Fluorescence is seen at the site of the tumor 48 hours after i.v. injection of hematoporphyrin derivative 2.5 mg/kg (right).*

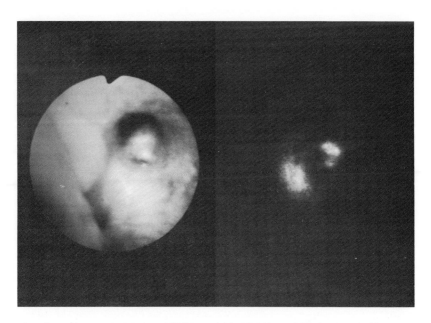

FIG. 6. *Photoradiation in a 50-year-old male (adenocarcinoma). Tumor invasion can be seen in the upper lobe bronchus (left). Fluorescence can be seen at the site of the tumor 48 hours after i.v. injection of hematoporphyrin derivative 2.5 mg/kg (right).*

Photoradiation therapy

Table 3 shows the therapeutic results of PRT in cases of lung cancer and of squamous-cell metaplasia. Complete tumor remission was obtained in 4 out of 5 early-stage cancers. In one early-stage case, partial remission was obtained and a second PRT procedure is scheduled in the near future. The periods since complete remission in the 4 cases were 1 year and 10 months, 10 months, 9 months and 2 months, respectively. These cases have been followed up intensively with fiberoptic bronchoscopy and cytological examinations. However, no recurrence has been recognized endoscopically so far, nor have tumor cells been obtained by brushing cytology. In 2 cases of severely atypical squamous-cell metaplasia the bronchial wall became smooth; no atypical cells were obtained after therapy.

Case 4 A 74-year-old male with cough, presented above as Case No. 2, was an early-stage case and a good candidate for surgery on the basis of his pulmonary and cardiac function etc., but he stubbornly refused

TABLE 3. *Therapeutic effects of hematoporphyrin derivative and photoradiation using an argon dye laser beam in lung cancer*

Stage	No. of cases	Complete remission	Significant remission	Partial remission
Early	5	4	1	0
Stage I	5	1	2	2
Stage II, III, IV	35	1	2	32
Total	45	6	5	34
Severe squamous-cell metaplasia	2	2	0	0
Total	47	8	5	34

T.M.C., Oct. 16, 1981.

surgery. Nevertheless, he did volunteer for PRT. The lesion was irradiated 3 times after a single i.v. injection of HpD 2.5 mg/kg body weight as follows: 150 mW $\times$ 20 min at 72 hours after injection, 150 mW $\times$ 10 min at 168 hours and 200 mW $\times$ 10 min at 240 hours. PRT was performed 3 times since this patient was only the second clinical case treated by PRT in our series, and we were afraid of possible local recurrence (Fig. 7). The tumor disappeared 3 days after the first PRT procedure. No tumor can be seen 1 year and 10 months after PRT (Fig. 8); no tumor cells have so far been obtained by brushing cytology.

Case 5 In a 59-year-old female presenting with cough and sputum, well-differentiated squamous-cell carcinoma cells were recognized on sputum cytology examination. However, her chest X-ray film was normal. A tumor was observed at the orifice of the right upper lobe bronchus, and the histological type was shown to be squamous-cell carcinoma. The case was early-stage, but inoperable due to her poor pulmonary function (VC 1530 ml, %VC 70.1 and %FEV$_{1.0}$ 58.2). PRT was therefore performed in April, 1981, 72 hours after i.v. injection of HpD 5.0 mg/kg body weight with a power output of 600 nm for 30 min (Fig. 9). The tumor disappeared 4 days after PRT. At present, 10 months after PRT, no tumor can be seen, and no tumor cells have been obtained by brushing cytology (Fig. 10).

Case 6 In a 50-year-old male with cough and a Brinkman index of 1200, squamous-cell carcinoma cells were obtained in a sputum cytology survey, although his chest X-ray was normal. Fiberoptic bronchoscopy

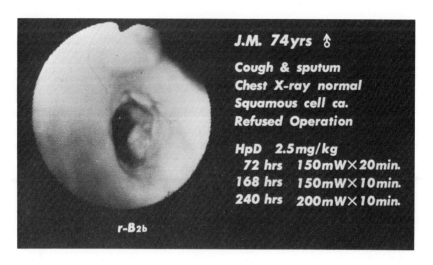

J.M. 74yrs ♂

Cough & sputum
Chest X-ray normal
Squamous cell ca.
Refused Operation

HpD 2.5mg/kg
72 hrs 150mW×20min.
168 hrs 150mW×10min.
240 hrs 200mW×10min.

r-B₂b

FIG. 7. *Fiberoptic bronchoscopic findings in the 74-year-old male case shown in Fig. 5. Photoradiation of the tumors in right B_2b was performed under the conditions shown on the right.*

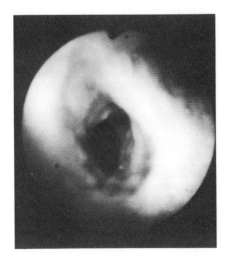

FIG. 8. *Fiberoptic bronchoscopic findings of the case shown in Fig. 7 after photoradiation therapy (PRT). No tumor can be seen 1 year and 10 months after PRT.*

64

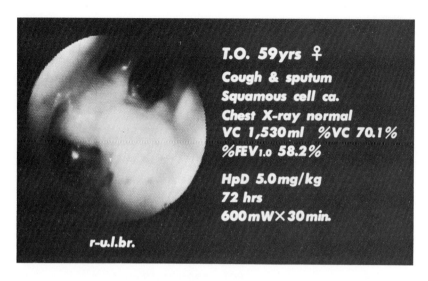

T.O. 59yrs ♀
Cough & sputum
Squamous cell ca.
Chest X-ray normal
VC 1,530ml   %VC 70.1%
%FEV1.0 58.2%

HpD 5.0mg/kg
72 hrs
600mW×30min.

r-u.l.br.

FIG. 9. *Fiberoptic bronchoscopic findings in a 59-year-old female. Photoradiation was performed on the tumor at the orifice of the right upper lobe bronchus (left) under the conditions shown on the right (squamous-cell carcinoma).*

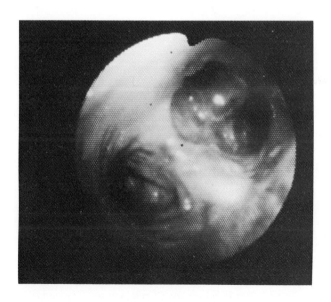

FIG. 10. *Fiberoptic bronchoscopic findings of the case shown in Fig. 9. No tumor can be seen 10 months after photoradiation.*

revealed invasion in the superior wall of the left upper division; biopsy showed the histological type to be well-differentiated squamous-cell carcinoma. The clinical stage was Stage Ia (T1, N0, M0) and PRT was performed using 300 mW power for 30 min. Two weeks after PRT, lobectomy of the left upper lobe was performed; neither tumor nor tumor cells could be seen in the superior portion of the orifice of the left upper division. However, the tumor was observed to have remained in left B_{1+2} (Fig. 11).

Y.A. 50y. Male Squamous cell carcinoma
Stage I

$\left(\begin{array}{l}\textbf{Positive sputum cytology}\\ \textbf{Negative chest X-ray findings}\end{array}\right)$

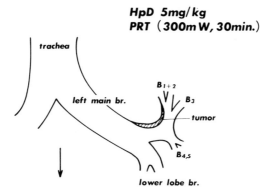

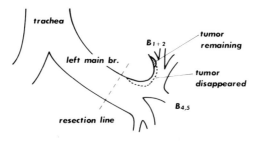

FIG. 11. *Schema of effects of photoradiation therapy (PRT) in a 50-year-old male with squamous-cell carcinoma. PRT of the tumor in the left upper division bronchus was performed with 300 mW power for 30 min (upper). The tumor in the superior portion of the orifice of the upper division disappeared, but the tumor in the superior portion of B_{1+2} remained (lower).*

Case 7 A tumor was observed at the bifurcation of the right lower division bronchus in a 55-year-old male with a negative chest X-ray but positive sputum. Features of squamous-cell carcinoma were observed on biopsy. Since intratumoral invasion was considered on the basis of the fiberoptic bronchoscopic findings and since he was also in Stage Ia (T1, N0, M0) clinically, lobectomy of the right middle and lower lobes was performed 2 weeks after PRT at 400 mW power for 25 min. The tumor and tumor cells at the bifurcation of the right lower division had disappeared completely, but remaining tumor was recognized in B_6 (Fig. 12).

S.N. 55y. Male Squamous cell carcinoma
Stage I
Positive sputum cytology
Negative chest X-ray findings

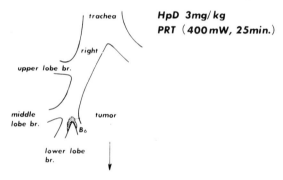

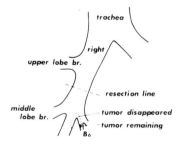

FIG. 12. *Effects of photoradiation therapy (PRT) in a 55-year-old male with squamous-cell carcinoma. The tumor in the right basal bronchus was irradiated with 400 mW power for 25 min (upper). Most of the tumor disappeared, but the tumor at B_6 remained (lower).*

Case 8 A 59-year-old male presented with atelectasis of the right upper lobe. The histological type of this case was well-differentiated squamous-cell carcinoma. Fiberoptic bronchoscopy revealed obstruction of the right upper lobe bronchus and invasion was observed in the trachea. The area of invasion received PRT for 20 min at 300 mW power. Seven days after PRT, the tracheal wall became smooth. Also, no tumor cells could be obtained from the site submitted to PRT. Sleeve resection of the right upper lobe was therefore performed 30 days after PRT. Detailed examination of the resected specimen revealed no tumor cells in the right upper lobe bronchus or bronchial stump in which invasion had previously been seen (Fig. 13). The patient is being followed up by bronchoscopy and cytology, but no recurrence has been observed 3 months after surgery.

Complications

Sensitivity to sunlight was observed to varying degrees in 88% of cases. In cases receiving 2 injections of HpD the color of the face became dark-brown. Obstructive pneumonia was observed in 2 cases due to a necrotic mass or exudate. Bronchial fistula developed in 2 inoperable Stage III

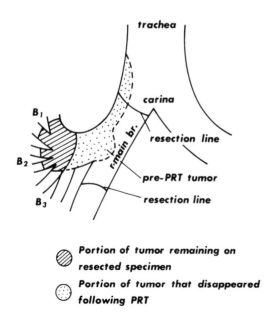

FIG. 13. *Schematic representation of a case receiving sleeve resection after photoradiation therapy of 300 mW for 20 min (squamous-cell carcinoma).*

cases of cancer located in the truncus intermedius after PRT, and one patient died from massive bleeding 3 months after PRT.

Discussion

Since HpD has an affinity for tumor tissue and remains longer in tumor than in normal tissue, several investigators have attempted tumor localization by observing HpD fluorescence (1, 2, 7). The first attempt to observe fluorescence endoscopically was made by Lipson and colleagues (17–19) using a mercury arc lamp to show fluorescence in the areas of invasion. Doiron and colleagues (3), Profio and colleagues (22) and Cortese and colleagues (2, 15) applied a photoradiation system using the flexible fiberoptic bronchoscope and succeeded in detecting one case of occult cancer which they were unable to localize by conventional fiberoptic bronchoscopy.

We employed a photoradiation system for tumor localization using a krypton ion laser beam which provides a coherent light of the most desirable wavelength for fluorescence excitation (9, 10, 12). In 35 cases of lung cancer, including 3 early-stage, central-type lung cancers, and also in 3 cases of severely atypical and 1 case of mildly atypical squamous-cell metaplasia, fluorescence was observed in all early cases and in severely atypical squamous-cell metaplasia. Fluorescence was seen in 29 out of 32 Stage I, II, III and IV lung cancer cases. Fluorescence could not be observed due to surface bleeding of the tumor, superficial necrotic tissue and submucosal growth, nor was it observed in 1 case of mildly atypical squamous-cell metaplasia. Thus tumor localization may be possible in cases undetectable by endoscopy, such as those with occult cancer, although all lung cancer cases in our series were diagnosed by fiberoptic bronchoscopy, even at an early stage. The possible role of squamous-cell metaplasia in the carcinogenetic process and the relationship between atypical squamous-cell metaplasia and invasive carcinoma remain to be elucidated. However, Drs. Saccomanno (23) and Nasiell (20) have recognized atypical squamous-cell metaplasia as a possible precancerous stage based on their retrospective cytological observations in lung cancer cases. The fact that fluorescence was observed in cases of severely atypical squamous-cell metaplasia is significant, in view of the difficulty of lesion localization by endoscopy, whereas no fluorescence was observed in the case of mildly atypical squamous-cell metaplasia. Of course, we do not suggest that the photoradiation system should be used for tumor localization in all stages of lung cancer, since most cases can be diagnosed by conventional endoscopy. The potential applications of photoradiation as a diagnostic method are: (1) lesion localization in a precancerous stage, (2) tumor localization in occult cancer, (3) detection of metastatic invasion of the trachea or bronchus apart from the primary lesion, (4) assessment of the extent of invasion to determine the site of bronchial transection, and (5) diagnosis of recurrent lesions in the bronchus after surgery.

Dougherty and colleagues (4, 5) introduced PRT for malignant tumors with a mercury arc lamp and laser beam following administration of HpD. However, the cases they treated with PRT were primarily in advanced stages. PRT for early-stage cancer, especially early-stage, central-type lung cancer, has been reported only by the present author and his colleagues (12–14). To clarify the therapeutic effectiveness and safety of PRT in early-stage lung cancer, we applied PRT with HpD in canine lung cancer induced successfully in large bronchi after a process producing progressively atypical squamous metaplasia (8, 11). We were able to confirm the safety and effectiveness of the system.

Complete tumor remission was obtained in 4 out of 5 cases of early-stage, central-type lung cancer, and in 2 out of 40 other lung cancer cases. Significant remission was obtained in 10% and partial remission in 85% of the other lung cancer cases. The post-PRT period is 1 year and 10 months, 10 months, 9 months and 2 months, respectively, in the early-stage cases; all cases are disease-free at present. Thus, we recognized the possible curative effect of PRT in early-stage lung cancer. Moreover, in 2 cases of severely atypical squamous-cell metaplasia, the atypia of the bronchial epithelium disappeared completely following PRT. This suggests the possible prophylactic value of PRT in precancerous lesions of the lung. Although significant or partial responses were obtained in Stage I and other stages, we should not expect to treat these cases only with PRT. However, one use of this method in Stage I and II cases is preoperative PRT (as described in Case 7), especially for cases of sleeve resection. In 3 Stage I cases resected after PRT, remaining tumor was observed at sites which could not be reached by the laser beam due to the angle of the bronchus. This requires improvement of the quartz fiber or perhaps intratumoral irradiation. Regarding intratumoral PRT by inserting the quartz fiber into the tumor, Dougherty and colleagues (6) used this method on animal tumors with a high rate of success. We have also used it in 2 human patients with intrabronchial tumor in whom our usual PRT method had been unsuccessful, and significant remission was obtained.

Among the complications of photoradiation, sensitivity to sunlight is not a significant side-effect, but massive bleeding after PRT is a critical problem. Cortese has presented cases succumbing to massive bleeding after PRT, and we have also recently experienced one case. In 2 cases, bronchial fistula developed after PRT, and extrabronchial growth was considered. We feel, therefore, that PRT should be performed carefully at low power for short periods and that due consideration should be given to the possible contraindications of PRT.

We consider the indications of PRT for lung cancer to be as follows: (1) prophylactic treatment of precancerous lesions, (2) curative therapy for inoperable early-stage, central-type lung cancer, (3) pretreatment for extended surgery, especially for sleeve resection, (4) pretreatment to decrease the required dose of radiation therapy, and (5) intratumoral PRT in inoperable cases.

Acknowledgements

The authors would like to express their appreciation to Dr. T.J. Dougherty for helpful advice and for kindly supplying HpD, and to Drs. E.G. King, G. Huth and E.C. Holmes and Mr. J.P. Barron for their cooperation.

References

1. Carpenter III, R.J., Ryan, R.J. and Sanderson, D.R. (1977): Tumor fluorescence with hematoporphyrin derivative. *Ann. Otol. Rhinol. Laryngol., 86,* 661–667.
2. Cortese, D.A., Kinsey, J.H., Woolner, L.B. et al. (1979): Clinical application of a new endoscopic technique for detection of in-situ bronchial carcinoma. *Mayo Clin. Proc., 54,* 635–641.
3. Doiron, D.R., Profio, E., Vincent, R.G. et al. (1979): Fluorescence bronchoscopy for detection of lung cancer. *Chest, 76,* 27–32.
4. Dougherty, T.J., Grindey, G.B., Fiel, R. et al. (1975): Photoradiation therapy. II. Cure of clinical tumor with hematoporphyrin and light. *J. nat. Cancer Inst., 55,* 115–121.
5. Dougherty, T.J., Lawrence, G., Kaufman, J.H. et al. (1979): Photoradiation in the treatment of recurrent breast carcinoma. *J. nat. Cancer Inst., 62,* 231–237.
6. Dougherty, T.J., Thoma, R.E., Boyle, D.G. and Weishaupt, K.R. (1981): Photoradiation therapy for treatment of tumors in pet cats and dogs. *Cancer Res., 41,* 401–404.
7. Gregorie Jr., H.B., Horger, E.D., Ward, J.L. et al. (1968): Hematoporphyrin derivative fluorescence in malignant neoplasma. *Ann. Surg., 167,* 820–828.
8. Hayata, Y., Kato, H., Chow, M. et al. (1977): Studies of the carcinogenetic process in experimental squamous cell carcinoma in canine lungs (in Japanese). *Jap. Soc. Chest Dis., 15,* 759–768.
9. Hayata, Y., Kato, H., Ono, J. et al. (1981): Fluorescence fiberoptic bronchoscopy for diagnosis of early stage lung cancer. In: *Recent Progress in Lung Cancer Research.* Editor: P. Band. Springer-Verlag, Berlin. In press.

10. Hayata, Y., Kato, H., Konaka, C. et al. (1981): Fiberoptic bronchoscopic laser photoradiation for tumor localization. *Chest,* in press.
11. Hayata, Y., Kato, H., Konaka, C. et al. (1981): Fiberoptic bronchoscopic photoradiation in experimentally induced canine lung cancer. *Cancer,* in press.
12. Hayata, Y., Kato, H., Konaka, C. et al. (1981): Hematoporphyrin derivative and laser photoradiation in the treatment of lung cancer. *Chest,* in press.
13. Hayata, Y., Oho, K., Kato, H. et al. (1981): Laser surgery (in Japanese). *Clin. Adult Dis., 11,* 87–93.
14. Hayata, Y., Kato, H., Ono, J. et al. (1981): Lung cancer and photoradiation (in Japanese). *Jap. Chest Clin., 40,* 383–388.
15. Kinsey, J.H., Cortese, D.A. and Sanderson, D.R. (1978): Detection of hematoporphyrin fluorescence during fiberoptic bronchoscopy to localize early bronchogenic carcinoma. *Mayo Clin. Proc., 53,* 594–600.
16. Lipson, R.L. and Baldes, E.J. (1960): The photodynamic properties of a particular hematoporphyrin derivative. *Arch. Derm., 82,* 508–516.
17. Lipson, R.L., Baldes, E.J. and Olsen, A.M. (1961): The use of a derivative of hematoporphyrin in tumor detection. *J. nat. Cancer Inst., 26,* 1–9.
18. Lipson, R.L., Baldes, E.J. and Olsen, A.M. (1961): Hematoporphyrin derivative: a new aid for endoscopic detection of malignant disease. *J. thor. cardiovasc. Surg., 42,* 623–629.
19. Lipson, R.L., Baldes, E.J. and Olsen, A.M. (1964): Further evaluation of the use of hematoporphyrin derivative as a new aid for the endoscopic detection of malignant disease. *Dis. Chest., 46,* 676–679.
20. Nasiell, M. (1966): Metaplasia and atypical metaplasia in the bronchial epithelium: a histopathologic and cytopathologic study. *Acta cytol., 10,* 421–427.
21. Profio, A.E., Doiron, D.R. et al. (1977): A feasibility study of the use of fluorescence bronchoscopy for localization of small lung tumor. *Phys. Med. Biol., 22,* 949–957.
22. Profio, A.E., Doiron, D.R. and King, E.G. (1979): Laser fluorescence bronchoscope for localization of occult lung tumors. *Med. Phys., 6,* 523–525.
23. Saccomanno, G., Archer, V.E., Auerbach, O. et al. (1972): Development of carcinoma of the lung as reflected in exfoliated cells. *Cancer, 33,* 256–270.
24. Sanderson, D.R., Fontana, R.S., Lipson, R.L. et al. (1972): Hematoporphyrin as a diagnostic tool: a preliminary report of new techniques. *Cancer, 30,* 1368–1372.

Hyperthermia for the treatment of cancer: biological, physical and clinical considerations

Norman M. Bleehen

Historical

Hyperthermia is not a new method of treatment for cancer. The use of heat has been advocated intermittently over the centuries. Hippocrates (400 B.C.) and Galen (200 A.D.) recommended hot irons to destroy tumours, but a variety of more sophisticated methods has been advocated during the past century. Currently, hyperthermia is used to describe treatment employing raised temperatures. These are usually between 41° and 45°C, maintained for periods of time varying from a few minutes to a few hours.

Clinical hyperthermia stems from the observations of Busch in 1866, who noted the disappearance of a histologically confirmed facial sarcoma after two attacks of erysipelas which were associated with high fever. Coley, in 1893, artificially induced repeated infections of erysipelas in patients with some success and subsequently developed his toxin. More selectively, Westermark, in 1898, used hot douches for patients with cancer of the cervix, with resultant arrest of haemorrhage and tumour regression.

Combined hyperthermia and radiation therapy was first advocated by Schmidt in 1909, who proposed the use of radiofrequency diathermy in combination with X-rays. Subsequently, Warren, in 1935, introduced whole-body heating with radiant heat and radiofrequency cabinets and also reported its combination with X-ray therapy (32). He carefully documented the responses of 32 patients with very advanced disease treated at 41.5°C for periods of up to 21 hours and subsequently repeated. In all except 3 patients, there was rapid symptomatic and sometimes objective improvement. He even observed possible synergism with deep X-ray therapy in one patient with ovarian cancer. However, he cautiously and sensibly concluded his paper with the statement that: 'It should be emphasized that no results approaching cure have yet been obtained by this procedure.'

73

Since these rather tentative and sporadic beginnings, a very considerable body of experimental work, particularly over the last decade, has been carried out to define biological mechanisms, which might permit design of optimal clinical therapy. Unfortunately, at present, our knowledge of the biology exceeds that of the physical methods available to induce satisfactory heat distributions in patients undergoing hyperthermia. In spite of this, many centres are now involved in experimental clinical hyperthermia.

This paper briefly reviews various aspects of our current knowledge about the subject. Particular emphasis is given to data relevant to lung cancer. It must be said, however, that these are sparse because primary bronchial carcinoma remains a very difficult site for current heating techniques. Only a few key-references are cited and the reader is recommended to consult several recent reviews for further details (11, 13, 14). Other relevant publications are reported in several recent symposia (5, 9, 26–28).

Biology

Very considerable advances have been made over the past decade in our understanding of the interaction of hyperthermia with experimental biological systems. As a result of this work, it is possible to forecast what may be its optimal usage either alone or in combination with ionizing radiation or anti-cancer drugs when applied to cancer therapy in man. Hyperthermia has been observed to kill cells when used alone and to interact with the cytotoxicity of X-rays and certain chemotherapeutic agents. This review will therefore assess in brief some relevant aspects of this experimental work, considering first the effects of heat alone and then those of its interaction with radiation and drugs. Detailed references are given in the reviews already cited, and in particular in Reference 11.

Heat alone

Cells in vitro from both animal and human origin show characteristic survival response curves when single exposures of heat are given for various temperatures or for different periods of time. The surviving fraction of cells is directly related to both the magnitude of the temperature and duration of exposure. An initial shoulder on the survival curve is followed by an exponential slope. With increasing temperatures, the size of the shoulder decreases and that of the slope becomes steeper. As an approximation, there is a doubling of cell-kill for every degree temperature rise above 42.5°C or at a constant temperature above 42.5°C for every doubling of the treatment time. However, there are considerable quantitative differences (10-fold or more) in the sensitivity to heat of the various cell lines so investigated.

Initial observations that malignant cells are more heat-sensitive than untransformed cells are now doubted, but this question remains finally to be resolved. Likewise, the early work indicated that hypoxic cells were very much more sensitive to heat than well-oxygenated ones, in direct contrast to the relative resistance of hypoxic cells to X-rays. This may still be true for some lines, but the phenomena are difficult to disentangle from other more significant effects such as pH variations. Thermal sensitivity is considerably increased at low pH, whether the cells are euoxic or hypoxic. Such a level of acidity might be expected within tumours as a result of their anaerobic metabolism.

An impoverished nutrient environment will also result in an enhanced hyperthermic cell-kill. Heat will kill cells at all stages of mitosis, but variations in sensitivity occur throughout the cell cycle. Cells in S-phase are very sensitive to heat, in contrast to their response at this stage to ionizing radiation when they are relatively resistant. Heat also results in greater mitotic delay than do X-rays for comparable levels of cell-kill. Thus there is marked heat-induced redistribution of cells through the cell cycle, an effect which can modify subsequent treatments with X-ray, drugs or even further heat.

The responses in vivo are similar to those described in vitro, with the added importance of local changes in the physiological environment such as pH, hypoxia, blood flow and physical parameters such as temperature gradients. These will frequently differ between tumour and normal tissues. The effect of pH in vitro is difficult to confirm in vivo, as direct measurements are technically difficult and open to question. When carried out with fine microelectrodes, measurements have usually shown a reduced pH in tumours. Experiments designed to decrease tissue pH either by prolonged ischaemia or glucose infusions have yielded results compatible with the general concept.

As has already been discussed, hypoxia *per se* may not increase thermal sensitivity, but will alter tissue pH and also thermal diffusion patterns. It is in the hypoxic zone that cells resistant to ionizing radiation are likely to occur. It is just these cells, which will be under adverse nutritional conditions with low pH and poor vascular perfusion, that should be most sensitive to thermal shock.

The response of normal tissues is obviously critical. The ultimate goal of hyperthermia should not be a demonstration of indiscriminate cell-kill, but a therapeutic gain resulting from a selective effect on tumours rather than normal tissues. The relationships between time and temperature seen with tumour cells in vitro and in vivo are also found with the many normal tissues, such as skin, cartilage or intestine, that have been investigated. In many instances, a difference in the effect slope is noted at increasing temperatures between 42° and 43°C. There is proportionately less killing as a result of the temperature increase than might have been expected from a linear relationship over the whole temperature range.

Cancer therapy with radiation or drugs usually employs fractionated courses and it is likely that hyperthermia will similarly require courses of repeated treatments. Tolerance to a subsequent heat-shock induced by a previous heat exposure is now well recognized in a variety of cell and tissue systems. This thermal tolerance may be demonstrated either by the diminished effect of prolonged single exposure (in excess of 3–4 hours) at temperatures below about 43.5°C. Such a situation occurs in techniques such as whole-body heating or regional perfusion. More relevantly, it can occur when two heat treatments are separated by a period of time, as in a fractionated course. The magnitude of this tolerance varies in the systems investigated, but can increase the heating time for an iso-effect of the second treatment by several-fold. The tolerance develops rapidly even after short treatment times and may be maximal at times ranging between 24 and 48 hours after the first heat-shock, and has largely disappeared by about 96 hours. In repeated courses, the degree of tolerance does not appear to be cumulative. Relevant clinical data are largely lacking, although there is some evidence of the existence of this phenomenon in man as well. It seems desirable, therefore, that clinical schedules should employ heat treatments separated by at least 3 or, better, 7 days, if thermal tolerance is not to occur.

Various mechanisms of thermal cytotoxicity have been proposed. No single explanation satisfies all the data and it is probable that several different molecular and physiological interactions are important. Molecular and cellular effects include: direct damage to DNA; either direct or indirect damage to RNA; effects on the cell membrane; labilization of the lysosomal membranes, with consequent intracellular release of lytic enzymes; and induction of specific heat-shock proteins possibly involved in the development of thermal tolerance.

In addition, there are the physiological and vascular effects, which will enhance cell killing. As already described, part of the therapeutic advantage of hyperthermia is thought to relate to differences between the blood flow in tumours and their surrounding normal tissue. The tumour vasculature is less uniform, with abnormal flow patterns which result in uneven perfusion and variable oxygen tension (TpO_2). This in turn is associated with alterations in tumour tissue pH, with an increased acidity. The tumour microvasculature appears to be particularly sensitive to hyperthermia. At temperatures below about 41°C, increased blood flow occurs in both tumours and normal tissues, whereas above 41°C, acute changes are seen in the tumour circulation with vessel dilatation followed by collapse and blood leakage. These effects, which are not seen in the normal tissue vessels, result in a further decreased TpO_2 and pH. In situ, hyperthermic tumour cell damage is then increased by the resultant ischaemia.

The above response pattern has been described in the laboratory work of several groups working with experimental tumour systems. Few measurements have been made in man and even less in lung cancer, although some of the advantageous effects of radiofrequency or microwave heating of deep-seated tumours, such as primary lung cancer, which have been reported were thought by the authors to be, at least in part, due to selective vascular effects (15, 19, 31). Higher tumour temperatures than in surrounding normal tissues have also been reported for superficial lesions with radiofrequency, for the same reasons (16).

Two groups of workers have measured vascular changes in secondary skin nodules from lung cancer. Mantyla (20) showed less blood flow in anaplastic and differentiated tumour nodules (including 7 squamous lung carcinomas) than in lymphomas. Bicher and his colleagues (3) reported on an extensive experimental and clinical study. In measurements on subcutaneous metastases in 15 patients (including 5 with squamous lung carcinoma), qualitatively similar changes in TpO_2, blood flow and pH were observed as in C3H mouse mammary tumour. The differences in effects above and below 41°C were also noted.

Heat with radiation

Heat and ionizing radiation have been demonstrated to act synergistically in a variety of model systems and in man. When this combination is tested in vitro, it is seen that there is a change in the slope of the cell-survival curve, indicating sensitization. In addition, there is frequently a reduction in the initial shoulder of the curve, indicating an impairment of the ability to accumulate and repair sublethal radiation damage. These effects will not necessarily be selective for malignant tissues. An additional effect in inhibiting the repair of potentially lethal damage may be therapeutically advantageous, as this form of repair is most likely to occur in nutritionally deprived and proliferation-limited cells.

A considerable body of in-vivo experimental work supports the view that similar effects are seen in both normal tissues and tumours when heat and radiation are combined concurrently. This will not therefore result in any therapeutic gain, unless the normal tissues can be protected by careful restriction of the treated volume or by external cooling, as described later, with some hyperthermia applicators. Initial data suggesting that thermal enhancement ratios were greater for some experimental tumours have been questioned on technical grounds, in particular because of the partial obstruction of the blood supply during the experiments.

The relative enhancement ratios, however, do differ when the heat and radiations are given separately in several animal model systems. Thus, with heat treatment given at 4 hours after irradiation, a greater response will be seen in tumour than normal tissue, with resultant therapeutic gain. Relevant clinical data are lacking, but many believe that separation of the radiation and heat treatments in a similar way is the best way to use the combination. Residual clonogenic but nutritionally deprived and hypoxic cells surviving the radiation will then be killed by the heat.

In spite of this theoretically based strategy, several clinical groups have treated with radiation and heat as closely together as possible. Differences in blood flow may well then protect the normal tissues by dissipating the heat more rapidly than in the tumour.

Heat and drugs

Hyperthermia will potentiate the cytotoxic effects of some chemotherapeutic agents. This is best documented with several of the alkylating agents, nitrosoureas and antibiotics. A list of the principal drugs demonstrated to interact in vitro is given in Table 1a. Other drugs or chemical agents have also been shown to interact under various conditions and are listed in Table 1b.

TABLE 1. *Drugs, toxicity of which is increased by heat*

a. Anti-cancer drugs

Cyclophosphamide	MeCCNU
Nitromin	Cisplatin
Melphalan	Adriamycin
MDMS	Bleomycin
Thiotepa	Macromycin
BCNU	Aclacinomycin
CCNU	Mitomycin

b. Other reagents

Alcohols	Polyamines
Amphotericin B	Thioglucose
AET	Misonidazole
Cysteamine	Local anaesthetics

There does not appear to be any single mechanism to explain the observed effects. The possible mechanisms involved are listed in Table 2. The most probable explanation for the enhancement of the effect of drugs such as the alkylating agents and nitrosoureas is thermodynamic, with increased drug activation and target interaction. The situation with antibiotics is more complex. Thus, increased intracellular concentration of adriamycin may result because of changes in cell membrane permeability, but no such increase is seen with bleomycin. With the latter drug, heat probably enhances its effect by inhibiting recovery from potentially lethal bleomycin damage.

Other drugs which are not inherently cytotoxic themselves may exhibit enhanced thermal cytotoxicity because of specific interactions. Thus, certain alcohols, local anaesthetics and amphotericin B probably interact at a cell membrane level. Others like misonidazole produce nitroduction products which interact with heat both directly and as a sensitizing agent when given before the hyperthermia.

Heat-induced drug tolerance has also been demonstrated, as with adriamycin, where prolonged heating may, in fact, reduce the cytotoxic effect of the drug. Thus, the interactions are complex and depend both on the type of drug and temperature employed. Useful enhancements are seen with alkylating agents at temperatures both above and below 42°C. In contrast, with antibiotics, temperatures in excess of 42°C are necessary, so that they are unlikely to be of value in whole-body techniques which are limited to a maximum of 42°C.

As with hyperthermia and radiation, the combination of heat and drugs does not appear to be a selective effect on tumours versus normal tissues. Indeed, the very scant experimental data suggest an increased enhancement of effect on normal critical tissues such as bone marrow. There is therefore a very real risk of enhanced toxicity with reduced (or negative) therapeutic gain when the combination is used in whole-body treatments. Likewise, local treatments may have increased morbidity, unless local cooling or vascular perfusion effects protect the normal tissue.

The potential advantages and disadvantages of the combination of hyperthermia and drugs are listed in Table 3.

TABLE 2. *Mechanisms of drug-hyperthermia interactions*

1. Thermodynamic increased interaction with target
2. Increased activation of drug
3. Increased drug access
4. Membrane and other interactions with previously inactive drugs
5. Effect on repair of sublethal or potentially lethal damage

TABLE 3. *Potential clinical advantages and disadvantages of the combination of hyperthermia and drugs*

Advantages
1. Hyperthermia-enhanced cytotoxicity of certain drugs
2. Spatial co-operation between the loco-regional treatment modality and the systemic drug treatment

Disadvantages
1. Increased normal tissue toxicity
2. Development of drug tolerance
3. Variations of drug concentrations due to perfusion differences between tumour and normal tissue
4. A theoretical risk of increased immunosuppression

TABLE 4. *Reported clinical uses of hyperthermia and drugs*

Drug	Heat by	Disease
Melphalan	Perfusion	Melanoma
Cyclophosphamide	Perfusion	Abdominal tumours
Adriamycin	Whole body	Various
	Local	Head and neck cancer
Bleomycin	Whole body	Lung, sarcomas
	Local	Head and neck cancer
CCNU, BCNU	Whole body	Melanoma

Other drugs which have been used include: actinomycin D, 5-fluorouracil, VP-16, vincristine, methotrexate, DTIC.

The current clinical uses reported for the combination of hyperthermia and drugs are listed in Table 4. The largest single usage has been with melphalan in limb perfusions for melanoma and sarcomas.

Predictive tests

There does not appear to be any particular group of experimental or clinical tumours intrinsically more responsive to hyperthermia than others. The individual clinical tumours treated have largely been selected because of their availability and feasibility for the heating techniques available. In the main, tests have been on superficial nodules, whilst deep-seated tumours, such as primary carcinomas of lung, have been particularly difficult to heat. The clinical results of such studies are discussed elsewhere in this review, but such empirical trials remain the only satisfactory test of likely response.

The possibility of laboratory tests predictive of clinical response has been discussed by Dickson and Suzangar (10) who demonstrated an inhibition of tissue respiration and/or glycolysis together with reduction of uptake of radiolabelled thymidine, leucine and uridine in tumour slices incubated at 37°C or 42°C for 4 hours, as compared with putative normal tissue controls which showed a much smaller effect. The results for lung tumours are compared with those from a variety of other tumours in Table 5. The lack of specificity of such tests on tumours isolated from their normal vascular environment reduces their likely value in clinical practice.

An alternative model is offered by the xenograft system. Human lung tumours frequently grow well in the immune-suppressed animal. For example, growth delay of the Co 1 poorly differentiated squamous lung carcinoma line implanted in nude mice following heat treatment has been demonstrated (12). Responses even for the same established cell line were very variable and it is unlikely that this technique will prove to be a practical one for individual patients, particularly as primary xenograft tumour takes are also so variable.

Summary of biological aspects in favour of clinical hyperthermia

It must be clear to the reader that hyperthermia is not ideally selective for cancer rather than normal tissues. However, certain of the phenomena already described require its serious consideration as an additional treatment modality, particularly as part of a combined modality therapy course with radiation and/or cytotoxic drugs.

The reasons for the potential clinical value of hyperthermia are summarized in Table 6. It can be seen that whilst hyperthermia itself may not be entirely satisfactory because of the problems already enumerated, in combination the treatment may at least be complementary and at some times even synergistic. It is for these biological reasons that clinical hyperthermia is of interest.

TABLE 5. *Biochemical response of tissue slices, after 4 hours at 42°C*

Tissue of origin	30% reduction in respiration and/or glycolysis	
	Tumour	Control
Lung	19/61	2/25
Others	35/100	2/49

Modified from Dickson and Suzangar (10).

TABLE 6. *Biological reasons for the potential clinical value of hyperthermia*

1. Tumour cells are at least as sensitive to heat as normal tissue cells
2. Hypoxic cells are at least as sensitive to heat as euoxic cells, in contrast to the reduced sensitivity of hypoxic cells to X-rays
3. Nutritionally deprived cells and cells at low pH, such as might be expected in the hypoxic portions of tumours, are more sensitive to heat than normal cells
4. Cells are more resistant to heat and X-rays at different stages in the cell cycle
5. Heat may enhance the effect of X-rays, but the time relationships are important
6. Heat may enhance the effect of some cytotoxic and other drugs, but dose and time relationships are important
7. Tumours may be selectively heated more than normal tissues with localized heating techniques because of their reduced vascular perfusion
8. The tumour microvasculature may be more sensitive to heat than the capillaries in normal tissues

Heating techniques

The major current difficulty besetting detailed clinical assessment of the value of hyperthermia for cancer therapy is that of the technology required for the delivery of heat to the target tumour volume. None of the current methods available, other than whole-body hyperthermia, which has its own problems, is very satisfactory for tumours situated at a depth of more than a very few centimetres. Methods for measuring the tissue temperature are invasive and interactive with the local vasculature. In the case of radiofrequency or microwave therapy, the temperature detectors may themselves be selectively heated. As already discussed, local changes in blood flow may alter heating patterns and these are not easily quantified.

None of the available techniques match up to the precision available with radiation therapy where tumour isodose distributions can be calculated because of predictable physical characteristics. The successful ionizing radiation technology sets standards by which hyperthermia requirements can be assessed. These are listed in Table 7.

Heating techniques are selected on the basis of their physical characteristics and the volume of tissue to be treated. Techniques are available for: whole-body, regional or more localized hyperthermia, employing direct heat from external sources; perfusion and infusion; and heat generated internally with radiofrequency, microwaves or ultrasound. It is the latter group which provides the methods most likely to be of value in the management of lung cancer. However, for the sake of completeness, a brief review is given of all the techniques.

TABLE 7. *Desiderata for hyperthermia techniques*

Equipment
1. Reliability, both electrical and mechanical
2. Reproducibility of output
3. Non-interactive thermometry
4. Ease of use by technicians (under supervision)
5. Power output sufficient for short heating times

Physical dosimetry
1. Should heat at depth
2. Should possess ability to overcome tissue inhomogeneities
3. Be possible to define the treatment volume
4. Thermometry to define minimum tumour temperatures and maximum normal tissue temperatures is required
5. Reasonable temperature homogeneity in the treatment volume is desirable

Clinical
1. Easily accepted by patient
2. As non-invasive as possible
3. Preferably not require anaesthesia
4. Produce therapeutic gain
5. Be cost-effective

TABLE 8. *Whole-body hyperthermia methods*

Method		Author (Ref. no.)
Cabinet	– radiant heat + diathermy	Warren (32)
	– hot air + radiofrequency	Pomp (25)
Bath	– wax + hot gas	Pettigrew (24)
Blanket	– heated water	Larkin (18)
Suit	– heated water	Bull (4)
Perfusion	– heated blood	Parks (23)

Whole-body hyperthermia

Pyrogen-induced hyperthermia, as used by Coley, is not currently considered practical. No agents have been identified which will reliably and safely raise the body temperature to a sufficient degree and precise duration. All methods of whole-body heating presently in use rely on heat transfer from external sources. These are listed in Table 8.

Stafford Warren (32) designed the cabinet method in a classical paper in 1935, and other modified versions have since been described. In this method, patients are placed in an enclosed chamber which can be heated by radiant heat or hot air; temperatures may be boosted by radio-frequency heating either to the whole patient or locally to the tumour. Temperatures in the range of 41–42°C may be achieved for periods of up to 21 hours. The Siemens cabinet is a present version of this method (25).

Immersion in hot water was used by Crile in 1968 and subsequently by Pettigrew who employs a hot wax bath to raise the body temperature (24). Patients are anaesthetized, wrapped in a polythene sheet and immersed in hot wax. Initially, the lungs were also used as a heat exchanger employing inhaled heated helium-oxygen mixtures, but this has been abandoned as both unnecessary and potentially hazardous because of the risk of fibrosing alveolitis. Once the desired temperature level is reached, it is maintained by opening the wax covering to allow cooling by evaporation of sweat.

Alternative methods for heat transfer have employed suits through which hot water is circulated (4) or heated blankets which are wrapped around the patient (18). These techniques are cumbersome and require anaesthesia. They may be associated with complications, although their incidence and type vary in the different reports. Generally, superficial burns are the major problem, but their incidence is still low, occurring in only a few percent of patients. Other complications that have been reported include disseminated intravascular coagulation, fibrosing alveolitis, pulmonary oedema, transient cardiac arrhythmias, hypotension and hepatic serum enzyme changes. The incidence of fatalities (circa 1%) has been remarkably low, in view of the types of patients treated.

A major limitation of the above methods is the rate at which heat can be transferred from the external source through the skin without causing burns. A build-up time of 90–120 min is usually required to reach a body temperature of 41.5–42°C, but this may be considerably longer. Somewhat more rapid heating, with the desired temperature being reached in 40–60 min, is achieved in the Siemens cabinet where the heat is supplied by a 27 MHz radiofrequency coil field electrode in its base.

An alternative method is that used by Parks and his colleagues (23). The patient's blood is warmed extracorporeally in a heat exchanger. There are 2 reservoirs, one for heated blood (48°C) and one for cooled blood (30°C), and appropriate mixing ensures rapid temperature control. The blood is then introduced through a dacron prosthesis inserted as a common femoral arterio-venous shunt. Temperatures are monitored at several sites. Oesophageal temperatures are reported to be raised to 41.5°C in as little as 22 min, but intravesical temperatures follow more slowly and may require a longer period of 15–45 min. These differences in temperature profiles emphasize how, even with whole-body heating, temperature homogeneity may be difficult to obtain. This is demonstrated by their observations in the treatment of a series of patients with lung cancer. Different temperature zones within the oesophagus could be identified, with regional differences of up to 1°C (23). These workers therefore specified their treatment temperatures as that measured inside the bladder.

The advantages and disadvantages of whole-body hyperthermia are listed in Table 9. A general systemic treatment is desirable when wishing to treat widely metastatic disease, possibly in combination with chemotherapy, although enhanced toxicity of the drugs on normal tissues may become a problem. Temperature measurement is relatively easy, although isolated core temperatures are not necessarily equivalent to those in tumours whose evaluation will still require invasive methods. The major disadvantages are probably: the low maximum temperature attainable (41.5–42°C); the lack of a protective temperature differential between tumour and normal tissues; and the cumbersome nature of the methods which usually require anaesthesia. In spite of these problems, some useful responses have been reported in patients with advanced disease using either single or several courses at 41.5–42°C for 1–4 hours.

Perfusion

Regional arterial perfusion has been used by several groups to treat a variety of diseases, notably melanoma and sarcoma of the limbs (6, 30). Sites at which the vascular supply is easily isolated are appropriate, particularly in the limbs, but there have also been brief reports of the treat-

---

TABLE 9. *Advantages and disadvantages of whole-body hyperthermia*

Advantages
1. Relative uniformity of temperature
2. Thermometry is easy
3. Systemic treatment suitable for both primary tumour and metastases
4. May be combined with chemotherapy

Disadvantages
1. No significant temperature differential between tumours and normal tissues
2. Temperature limited to 42°C
3. Slow and complicated and usually requires anaesthesia
4. Systemic toxicity of its own
5. Enhanced toxicity when combined with chemotherapy

---

ment of brain and abdominal tumours. As with the whole-body perfusion, blood is heated extracorporeally; because the region is isolated, high-dose chemotherapy may also be employed simultaneously without major risk of general systemic toxicity.

The regional temperature can be raised to 41.5–43.5°C for periods of up to 6 hours and treatments may be repeated. Treatment, temperature and duration, region isolated, and whether or not cytotoxic drugs are also used, vary according to author. Sometimes local X-ray therapy is also added. To overcome the difficulty in maintaining satisfactory steady-state temperatures, due to physical differences between tumour and normal tissues, Cavaliere and his colleagues (6) wrapped the perfused limbs with warm rubber blankets. This was largely successful, except with osteogenic sarcomas where presumably the osseous circulation remained independent of the perfusion technique.

The recorded complications largely depend on the experience of the group employing the techniques, but in general they are acceptable. The results of around 1000 patients reported in 10 different series indicate a mortality rate due to the procedure of around 3% and a similar percentage requiring limb amputation as a result of major necrosis. Both complication rates are regarded by the authors of the largest series to have been reduced in their latest patients. The only other common complication is that of tissue necrosis requiring surgical debridement, which occurs in 1–2% of patients.

Although this method has its enthusiastic advocates, it has not been used for the management of lung cancer because of its obvious technical difficulties.

Intracavitary infusions

Local heating of body cavities containing tumours has been attempted by a few authors. The principal site so treated has been the bladder. The bladder temperature is raised by perfusion with fluid at temperatures between 44° and 82°C for times ranging from 240 to 5 min depending on the temperature employed. The results have been disappointing, because the major effects seen have always been damage to the normal mucosa with ensuing necrosis, haemorrhage and contracture.

Hyperthermic peritoneal lavage has been used in conjunction with chemotherapy in the treatment of a few patients with widespread disease from carcinoma of the ovary and pancreas. Temperatures of around 52°C were maintained for 30 min during repeated treatments. Results are difficult to assess and the methods are not likely to be relevant to the management of lung cancer.

The physical and biological effects of ultrasound are complex and include both non-thermal and thermal effects. The latter are due to cavitation, acoustic streamlining and radiation force. Their value in cancer therapy is thought largely to depend on thermal effect. An historical review of the subject is presented by Kremkau (17), whilst more detailed physical aspects are reviewed elsewhere (14, 28). Preliminary clinical results using ultrasound have been reported (21, 27, 28).

Ultrasound is generated from a piezo-electric transducer which, when activated by a high-frequency voltage, produces pressure waves. This mechanical energy will propagate through air and soft tissues as longitudinal waves, which generally become attenuated with the production of heat. Both longitudinal and transverse waves may occur in bone and attenuation is more rapid. Data on the attenuation coefficients of tissues in man are sparse and will vary according to their frequency which is usually in the range of 0.5–5 MHz. Over this frequency range, penetration depths, which are defined as the depth at which the incident power density is reduced to approximately 14% of incident for ideal phantom models, is 12 and 1.2 cm in muscle, 20 and 2.0 cm in fat, and 3 and 0.09 cm in bone for frequencies of 0.5 and 5 MHz, respectively. In air, ultrasound attenuates very rapidly and hence transducers are coupled to the body surface with an aqueous gel, or de-gassed water. Consequently, air cavities within body and particularly in the lungs reduce the potential of therapeutic ultrasound in such regions. In addition to attenuation on passing through tissues, reflection of ultrasound from interfaces also causes changes in energy distributions.

The short wavelengths of ultrasound in the soft tissues are of the order of 0.3–0.03 cm over the frequency range 0.5–5 MHz. As the dimensions of the minimum volume treated are directly dependent on the wavelength, ultrasound has the advantage of enabling treatment of smaller volumes of tissue than are possible with the relatively longer wavelengths of microwave and radiofrequency radiation. The maximum surface area treated depends on the size of the transducer crystal available (currently about 5 cm diameter).

Single transducers may therefore be used to heat superficial tumours in the skin and head and neck region, but field size and attenuation limit treatment of larger tumours at depth and differential heating of bone may also then cause problems. The lack of selective heating of fat in subcutaneous tissues is a definite advantage over capacitive radiofrequency heating.

The small angle of divergence of the ultrasound beam from a transducer permits the construction of focussed bowl transducers. The focal volume from such transducers is likely to be smaller than the tumour volume, a difficulty which may be overcome by scanning the transducer over the target volume. Alternative methods use ultrasound lenses or mirrors to focus the beam or use crossed beams of several plane transducers. Better temperature profiles at depth are likely to result from phased arrays of transducer elements activated in sequence. In an annular array, concentric ring sources may focus the beam at any desired point along the treatment axis.

An additional advantage of ultrasound is the absence of interaction with temperature-measuring devices. Other properties of ultrasound include its imaging potential and plans to employ an imaging transducer in hyperthermic arrays have been proposed, to allow the treatment volume to be visualized. More speculative, but theoretically feasible, is the non-invasive measurement of temperature which utilizes the observation that the velocity of sound is a function of the temperature.

The practical advantages and disadvantages of ultrasound hyperthermia are summarized in Table 10. The problem raised by attenuation in bone and air and reflection at their interfaces probably make it an unlikely candidate as a method for the treatment of primary lung cancer, although for other soft tissue sites it holds much promise.

Non-ionizing electromagnetic radiation

Non-ionizing electromagnetic (EM) waves are currently favoured methods for local heating. Heating results from ionic movements generated by the electric fields and the rotation of polar molecules in the alternating fields. The extent of the interactions will depend on the frequency of the EM radiation and the electrical properties of the tissues. The latter are normally called dielectric properties which may be expressed by mathematical functions. The details of this are beyond the scope of this review, but the electrical properties of tissues will largely depend on their water content. Tissues may be grouped into those with high water content, such as muscle, skin and visceral organs, and those, such as bone and fat, which have a low value. These groups of tissues will be differentially heated by radiation at a given frequency, while different variations may occur at other frequencies. It is these properties and the attenuation of the EM radiation with depth in tissue which determine their usefulness for the induction of local hyperthermia. The very different dielectric properties of most temperature detectors, such as metallic thermocouples, makes their use with EM radiation both difficult and prone to error.

Further details of EM methods of heating are given in recent reviews (13, 29) and their contained references and the recent Hyperthermia Conference Symposia listed in the introduction (5, 9, 26–28).

TABLE 10. *Comparison of radiation heating methods*

Radiation	Advantages	Disadvantages
Ultrasound	Best for focussing with good depth dose from single and multiple arrays up to 15 cm. Fat not preferentially heated. Non-interactive with thermometers. Possible use for imaging and thermometry	Bone heating and reflections. Air/tissue interface reflections. Coupling medium required. Not suitable for lung cancer
Radiofrequency capacitive	Heats large volumes at fair depths, especially with multiple applicators. Skin cooling possible. Suitable for lung cancer	Superficial fat and skin excessively heated – may be helped by skin cooling. Heating pattern unpredictable. Interacts with metal thermometers
Radiofrequency inductive	Heats large volumes at depth, especially with multiple applicators. Little excess heating of skin and fat. Possible for lung cancer	Heating pattern unpredictable and not well localized. Interacts with metal thermometers.
Radiofrequency implants	Volumes specifically localized	Invasive and limited by accessibility
Microwaves	Large volumes heated and good depth of doses possible with multiple applicators or phased arrays. Can be used in cavities with co-axial applicators. Possible for lung cancer	Limited depth dose from single applicators. Interacts with metal thermometers. Stray microwaves may need shielding

Radiofrequency　Radiofrequency EM radiation in the frequency range of 0.5–30 MHz has been used to heat tissues since the turn of the century. Initially, frequencies of the order of 1 MHz were used in long-wave diathermy, but these carried a high risk of superficial burns, so that higher frequencies were subsequently selected. Currently, 13.56 and 27.12 MHz are employed as accepted ISM (Industrial, Scientific and Medical) frequencies for what is known as short-wave diathermy. Their allocation for purposes other than radiocommunication permits their use in unscreened areas, whereas with other frequencies electrical screening may be necessary.

Radiofrequency heating is usually carried out by 2 principal methods employing either capacitive or inductive coupling of the EM energy. Capacitive coupling employs pairs of metallic electrodes, connected to the radiofrequency generator, between which the electrical fields produce a current density proportional to the power input, but also related both to the size of the electrodes and to variations in the distance between them. Compared with underlying muscle and soft tissues, subcutaneous fat has a high resistance, dissipates heat less well because of its poor thermal conductivity and vascular perfusion, and may be exposed to a high current density because of its proximity to the surface. All these factors increase the danger of excessive heating of subcutaneous fat when using capacitive coupling. This risk is usually overcome by cooling the skin beneath the electrodes, which should have dimensions at least as large as the area of the tissue to be heated in order to avoid excessive superficial current density. The use of saline solution, with a resistivity matched to tissues, in a flexible bag between the electrodes and skin permits better contour matching and reduces the risks of superficial overheating and resultant burns. The use of more than one pair of electrodes in a cross-fire also helps to obtain uniform heating.

Treatments using capacitive radiofrequency techniques have been used by Le Veen and colleagues (19) and by Storm and colleagues (31). Both use 13.56 MHz in their specially designed equipment which have the potential for cross-fire techniques. The 'Magnetrode' (31) also can be used with ring electrodes for inductive coupling. Several other groups have also either constructed their own equipment and electrodes or used commercially available short-wave diathermy machines. It is possible that sufficient heating at depth in the thorax may occur with multiple applicators.

Inductive coupling occurs in tissues close to a coil carrying a radiofrequency current. The magnetic field included by the alternating current in the coil results in a flow of current in the tissues. This will be greater in muscles and viscera with a high water content than in fat and bone, an advantage over capacitive coupling. However, flat coil applicators with up to 3 wire rings, known as pancake coils, will still only heat relatively superficially to a depth of a few centimetres. The heat energy deposited in the plane of the coil is also not very uniform. This may partially be overcome by the use of pairs of coils connected in series or more complex ring arrangements around the segments of the patient to be treated, as in the Magnetrode (31).

Storm and his colleagues use 13.56 MHz for inductive heating by the Magnetrode coils and claim selective heating at considerable depths in the thorax and abdomen suitable for the treatment of primary lung cancer (31). The pancake coils of the type used by Kim and Hahn (16) for inductive heating at 27.12 MHz are not really suitable for such deep-seated tumours, because of their poor depth dose.

Two other techniques for heating by radiofrequency have been proposed. In the first, localized current fields may be produced when electrical currents of low frequency (0.1–10 MHz) pass between electrodes either in superficial contact or implanted in the tissue volume to be treated. Such a technique has been proposed for viscera, such as oesophagus or colon, using large external electrodes together with an endocavitary cylindrical one. Alternatively, needle electrodes may be inserted as arrays into more superficial tumours in a technique reminiscent of radium needle implants. The second new technique relies on the selective heating of metallic seeds or particles implanted into the tumours. Both these techniques are invasive and the latter has the additional disadvantage of requiring high-power output and a permanent foreign-body implant. However, there may be some potential for the management of lung cancer, as the electrodes may be suitably positioned either in the lumen of the oesophagus adjacent to the tumour at the time of thoracotomy.

The advantages and disadvantages of radiofrequency hyperthermia are summarized in Table 10.

Microwaves Electromagnetic (EM) radiations in the frequency range 300–300,000 MHz (0.3–300 GHz) are known as microwaves. In general, the ISM frequencies available are 434, 915 and 2450 MHz, although not in all countries. Unlicensed frequencies can only be used in shielded rooms. Depth of penetration decreases with increasing frequency. Energy absorption is greatest in wet tissues such as skin, muscle and tumour and much less in fat and bone. At 2450 MHz the penetration depth in wet tissues is about 2 cm, whilst in bone and fat it is approximately 3.5 and 30 cm.

In general, direct contact applicators are used. The design of those in use may be complex, as loading with suitable dielectric materials, ridging of the base and overall shape will all determine the uniformity of energy distribution delivered. With single applicators, maximum heating will always occur near to the surface, that is in skin. It is for this reason that most surface applicators have built-in cooling devices to reduce the skin temperature, unless the requirement is to treat very superficial tissue.

Large volumes are easily heated by microwaves, but because of their limited penetration, even at the lower frequencies, heating at depth is not possible with single external applicators. Opposed applicators can improve the temperature distribution but still not achieve adequate central heating at depths equivalent to the thorax in man. Further benefit may be obtained by the use of multiple applicators. However, to date, thermal profiles have not been adequately assessed with this type of equipment.

The recent development of synchronous phased arrays of applicators has been shown theoretically, and in phantoms, to produce excellent heating at depths suitable for mid-thoracic or abdominal treatment. Some precision in the size of the heated volume and its localization may be obtained by appropriate selection and timing of the arrays. Such equipment is already in commercial development (29) using arrays of 915 MHz generators and is under clinical trial in several centres. Sophisticated computerized control systems are required, since the power output can be altered by interactions between the microwave and the tissue being treated.

A more direct method of delivering microwave energy is by means of co-axial applicators which can be used over a wide range of frequencies. These may be of sufficiently small diameter to be implanted directly into tumours or inserted into cavities such as the oesophagus, vagina and cervix.

The advantages and disadvantages of microwave hyperthermia are listed in Table 10. In summary, none of the techniques listed in this section is in any way ideal. Compromises in thermal profiles and volumes treated have to be accepted until the development of better techniques. Also, it is unlikely that any one method will be suitable for all tumours.

Thermometry   The very close relationship between the degree of thermal damage inflicted on tissue and the temperatures and time to which these tissues are exposed makes accurate thermometry essential. Theoretical calculation on the basis of physical parameters, perhaps checked by measurements in phantoms, is insufficient because of the variations in physical conditions such as vascular perfusion which may occur from day to day. The problems involved and some of the possible solutions are reviewed in detail elsewhere (7, 8).

All current methods are invasive, in that the detector needs to be placed within the site of measurement. Apart from the technical difficulties in placing the detectors in situ, especially in poorly accessible tumours, discomfort to the patient may be considerable when several probes are required, as is usual. There will also be the need to repeat measurements at successive treatments. Tumours of the lung clearly present major difficulties in this respect. Techniques of implanting fine polythene tube guides which can take repeated insertions of thermocouples have been described for more superficial tumours, but do not seem very appropriate in the thorax.

There are also questions to be raised about the relevance of the temperatures measured by these implanted detectors. Firstly, they are likely themselves to alter the local blood flow because of their finite dimensions. Perhaps more importantly is the interaction, already mentioned, of detectors with dielectric constants dissimilar to that of tissue with EM radiations. Thus, metallic wires, contained in thermocouples, will themselves also become selectively heated and additionally may disturb the EM field patterns.

Various methods are used to overcome these physical difficulties. Thus, implanted thermocouples should be as fine as possible and their long axis perpendicular to the incident field if possible. Non-perturbing probes include optical fibres with liquid crystal detectors, birefringent crystals or small semiconductors.

Non-invasive thermometry with conventional thermometers is not nearly precise enough. However, the possibility of using ultrasound attenuation, which is dependent on temperature, in computerized reconstruction tomography, has already been mentioned and is being investigated. Ideally, suitable techniques should give continuous non-interactive measurements from a close grid of locations in both tumour and heated normal tissue to an accuracy of within 0.1°C. This we are as yet unable to do.

Clinical experience

So far, this review has summarized in general the current status of the biological and physical basis on which the practice of clinical hyperthermia may be built. The major problems involved in the physical techniques should be overcome by research and development. The physiological variations are less predictable and may well prove more difficult, as they are often individual to the patient and his tumour. In spite of this, the potential biological advantages in favour of hyperthermia as a treatment modality have initiated a considerable number of clinical trials. This section reviews the status of these trials, with particular reference to lung cancer. Comprehensive analysis is not possible as methods and details reported vary between series which may include from 1 to more than 100 patients. It is convenient to review these results on the basis of the heating method employed.

Whole-body hyperthermia

Approximately 600 patients are reported in the literature at the time of review (mid-1981). These have been variously treated with heat alone or in combination with radiation or cytotoxic drug therapy. The drugs used have not always been of the functional type likely to have interacted with heat on the basis of laboratory evidence. Because of the experimental nature of the treatments, studies have largely been Phase 1 and 2 investigating toxicity more than tumour responses, as patients have usually had advanced disease not responsive to conventional treatments.

The collated results from 8 sources, in terms of response rates, are presented in Table 11, together with a more detailed analysis of those patients with carcinoma of the bronchus on whom details have been reported. The tumours include both primary and secondary disease and a variety of histological types. The paucity of numbers makes detailed conclusions impossible. Amongst the non-bronchial tumours, it is of interest that diseases classically responding poorly to drugs and radiation seem to respond as well to heat as those tumours which are more sensitive to radiation and drugs. Thus responses in bone sarcomas, melanoma and bowel tumours are reported with reasonable frequency. Unfortunately, responses are usually transient and long-term control has not usually been reported.

Results reported for lung cancer (2, 18, 22–24) are collated in Table 11. Larkin (18) induced hyperthermia with a heated water blanket and reports objective responses in 6/22 patients with lung cancer, but details of heat, histological type, drug and radiation treatments and duration of responses for this group of his patients are not given. Parks and his colleagues (23) induced systematic hyperthermia with extracorporeal heating. A total of 97 treatments each averaging 5 hours at 41.5°C were given to 25 patients, 23 of whom had previously failed on radiation or chemotherapy. Only 7 patients received hyperthermia alone; the majority received it in combination with chemotherapy (cyclophosphamide, adriamycin or cyclophosphamide with BCNU). Objective regressions

TABLE 11. *Tumour responses in whole-body hyperthermia*

Disease and treatment	Number of patients	Total response (CR + PR)	CR
All diseases	588	185 (31%)	18/295 (6%)
Bronchus*			
All treatments	66	30 (45%)	7 (9%)
H	5	2	0
H + C	47	19	3
H + R	8	4	1
H + R + C	6	5	3

* Treatment: heat (H); chemotherapy (C); radiation (R).
Collated from literature in 1981.

were seen in 13/25 patients with 3 complete responses. Of 12 patients at risk for 4 months or more, 4 had stable regressed disease at 20, 13, 8 and 7 months after hyperthermia. Neumann and his colleagues (22) reported on 14 patients with lung cancer treated in the Siemens cabinet either combined with radiotherapy and/or chemotherapy. Histological types included 2 undifferentiated, 6 squamous-cell and 6 small-cell carcinoma. There were 11 responders (including 6 CR) of which 5 were without tumour progression 4–15 months later. Analysis of the effect of hyperthermia is difficult because of the combination with the other effective modalities.

These and the other groups are continuing to investigate the place of whole-body hyperthermia in lung cancer. It is likely that the most valuable methods will be in combination with radiation therapy to the primary together with chemotherapy.

Perfusion

Techniques and results of whole-body hyperthermia by perfusion have already been discussed, as have the methods for regional hyperthermia. Regional treatment has been used for tumours of limbs, in particular melanoma and soft tissue and bone sarcomas (6, 30). The results, summarized in Table 12, are difficult to assess because of the absence of suitable controls, although favourable responses are reported.

There are no reports of the use of regional perfusion in lung cancer. Because of the obvious technical difficulties of access to the appropriate tumour vasculature, it seems unlikely that this method will be of much practical use for this disease.

Local hyperthermia by non-ionizing radiation

Most clinical hyperthermia currently employs local heating of the

TABLE 12. *Regional hyperthermia by perfusion*

Region	Tumour	Number of patients	Number of series	% 5-year survival*
Limb perfusions	All reported	856	9	
	Melanoma	452	5	59–88
	Soft tissue sarcoma	150	2	20–62
	Bone sarcoma	74	2	60
Brain	Glioma	5	1	
Abdomen	Various diseases	25	1	

* For selected stages and crude or actuarial survival.
Collated data from literature (6/81).

tumour volume by radiofrequency, microwaves or ultrasound. Depth-dose considerations already discussed have limited their usefulness and only very recently are techniques becoming available which may be suitable for the management of primary lung cancer. The presence of lung and bone seriously impedes the induction of uniform tumour temperatures. However, selective heating has been described as a consequence of reduced tumour cooling resulting from poor vascular perfusion.

The bulk of current data has been accumulated in the treatment of superficial skin nodules in patients with advanced disease. These have confirmed the biological effects observed in experimental models. Single or fractionated treatments for periods of 15 min to 2 hours at 41–50°C have been used, frequently with skin cooling in an attempt to reduce damage to normal tissue. A variety of histological types has been treated and no particular response sensitivities identified. Results vary and range from complete responses for several months or years to transient partial responses of a few weeks to non-responders.

Le Veen and his colleagues (19) have reported on the use of 13.56 MHz capacitive heating on 6 patients with lung cancer. Subsequent histological examination showed extensive tumour necrosis.

Kim and Hahn (16) employed a commercially available, inductive radiofrequency diathermy machine. They heated superficial tumours (principally melanoma and mycosis fungoides) to 41–43.5°C for 30–90 min and combined these treatments with radiotherapy. Some of the nodules received radiotherapy alone. A considerably improved response rate was observed when both treatments were given together, as seen in Table 13. Some enhancement of the radiation-induced skin reaction was seen, but usually only when the areas treated were scarred, had been skin-grafted primarily or when fractionated radiation in excess of 5 Gy per session were used and the heat was given before the radiation.

Arcangeli and his colleagues (1) treated tumour-involved lymph nodes in the head and neck region with 500 MHz microwaves. In a complex randomization protocol, some received multidose X-ray fractions per

TABLE 13. *Hyperthermia by 27.12 MHz inductive radiofrequency for superficial tumours*

Treatment	Total number of patients	Tumour response	
		Complete (CR)	% CR
Radiation	49	12	26%
Radiation + heat	54	42	78%

Data from Kim and Hahn (16).

day, others chemotherapy with adriamycin or bleomycin. Radiotherapy or chemotherapy was given either alone or in combination with hyperthermia. Their results, in terms of responses at the end of treatment, are summarized in Table 14. The total numbers involved are relatively small. However, for the 2 chemotherapy regimes taken together, the responses of those also receiving heat is significantly better ($P < 0.01$) than those on drug alone.

Capacitive radiofrequency at 13.56 MHz has been used by Herbst and Sauer (15) in a series of 62 patients including 8 with bronchial carcinoma and 5 with metastases in the lungs. Skin cooling was used. Heating cycles of 45–60 min thought to raise the tumour temperature (usually unmonitored) to around 45°C were followed immediately afterwards by 2 Gy of X-rays. Radiotherapy was given 5 days a week to total doses of up to 60 Gy with hyperthermia for 4 and subsequently 2–3 times a week. Analysis of the significance of the hyperthermia is difficult because of the combination with X-rays and the method of scoring the response. However, 6/8 bronchial carcinoma patients are reported to have shown a good response and 2/5 of those with lung metastases.

Inductive radiofrequency heating at 13.56 MHz, as reported by Storm and his colleagues, has been claimed to provide selective tumour heating in the thorax with marked responses (31). In a subsequent report, crossfire heating at ≥45°C was claimed to produce 'benefit' in 8/37 lung tumours (27).

Ultrasound heating has so far been used mainly for the treatment of superficial lesions (21). In general, the role of ultrasound hyperthermia remains to be assessed. For the reasons listed in the Methods section, it

TABLE 14. *Hyperthermia by 500 MHz microwaves for malignant head and neck nodes either alone or in combination with multidose radiotherapy or chemotherapy*

Responders at the end of treatment		
Heat + drug		Drug only
ADM	9/20	4/11
BLM	11/11	6/11
Total*	20/21	10/22
Heat + radiotherapy		Radiotherapy only
Complete response	17/25	12/25
Partial response	4/22	8/25

* $P < 0.01$
Data from Arcangeli and colleagues (1).

is only likely to be of considerable value at sites other than the thorax and upper abdomen and therefore not suitable for primary lung cancer.

Clinical conclusions

The clinical results of hyperthermia in cancer management currently available are largely anecdotal. Documented responses have been obtained, even in primary lung cancer. However, in general, the studies must largely be regarded as Phase I feasibility and toxicity investigations. Further assessment of the practical role in the management of lung cancer awaits the improved techniques now coming into practice. Indeed, by the time of the III World Conference on Lung Cancer in May, 1982, 9 months after the collation of this review, there may well be more exciting results.

Summary

1. Hyperthermia at temperatures in excess of 41 °C for intervals ranging from minutes to hours will destroy both clinical and experimental tumours for a variety of reasons.
2. Normal tissue effects limit the heat dose possible, but physiological differences between tumours and normal tissues may result in therapeutic gain.
3. Hyperthermia may interact with both ionizing radiation and cytotoxic drugs with therapeutic benefit.
4. The methods available for clinical hyperthermia include a variety of whole-body techniques. Regional heating may be achieved by perfusion; local heating is possible with radiofrequency, microwaves and ultrasound.
5. Each of the available methods has major limitations and in particular when applied to the management of primary lung cancer because of its situation in the thorax surrounded by air and bone.
6. Adequate measurement of tumour temperatures is currently both inaccurate and difficult.
7. Current early clinical results in a large variety of tumours, including a few lung cancers, suggest that further investigation into the value of hyperthermia in the management of lung cancer should continue.

References

1. Arcangeli, G., Cividalli, A., Lovisolo, G., Mauro, F., Creton, G., Nervi, C. and Pavin, G. (1980): Effectiveness of local hyperthermia in association with radiotherapy or chemotherapy: comparison of multimodality treat-

ments on multiple neck node metastases. In: *Proceedings, 1st Meeting of the European Group of Hyperthermia in Radiation Oncology*, pp. 257–265. Editors: G. Arcangeli and F. Mauro. Masson, Milan.

2. Barlogie, B., Corry, P.M., Yip, E., Lippman, L., Johnston, D.A., Khalih, K., Tenczynski, T.F., Reilly, E., Lawson, R., Dosik, G., Rigor, B., Hankenson, R. and Freireich, E.J. (1979): Total body hyperthermia with a resultant chemotherapy for advanced human neoplasms. *Cancer, 39*, 1481–1489.

3. Bicher, H.I., Hetzel, F W., Sandhu, T.S., Frinak, S., Vaupel, P., O'Hara, M.D. and O'Brien, T. (1980): Effects of hyperthermia on normal and tumour microenvironment. *Radiology, 137*, 523–530.

4. Bull, J.M., Lees, D., Schuette, W., Whang-Peng, J., Smith, R., Bignum, G., Atkinson, E.R., Gottdiener, J.S., Gralnick, R., Shawker, T.H. and DeVita, V.T. (1979): Whole body hyperthermia: a phase-I trial of a potential adjuvant to chemotherapy. *Ann. intern. Med., 90*, 317–323.

5. Streffer, C., Van Beuningen, D., Dietzel, F., Rottinger, E., Robinson, J.E., Scherer, E., Seeber, S. and Trott, D.R. (Eds.) (1978): *Cancer Therapy by Hyperthermia and Radiation*, pp. 3–344. Urban and Schwarzenberg, Baltimore–Munich.

6. Cavaliere, R., Moricca, G., DiFilippo, F., Caputo, A., Monticelli, G. and Santori, F.S. (1980): Heat transfer problems during local perfusion in cancer treatment. *Ann. N.Y. Acad. Sci., 335*, 311–326.

7. Cetas, T.C. and Connor, W.G. (1978): Thermometry considerations in localised hyperthermia. *Med. Phys., 5*, 79–91.

8. Christensen, D.A. (1979): Thermal dosimetry and temperature measurements. *Cancer, 39*, 2325–2327.

9. Milner, J.W. (Ed.) (1979): Proceedings, Conference on Hyperthermia in Cancer Treatment, 1979. *Cancer Res., 39, Part 2*, 2235–2340.

10. Dickson, J.A. and Suzangar, M. (1976): A predictive in vitro assay for the sensitivity of human solid tumours to hyperthermia (42°C) and its value in patient management. *Clin. Oncol., 2*, 141–155.

11. Field, S.B. and Bleehen, N.M. (1979): Hyperthermia in the treatment of cancer. *Cancer Treat. Rev., 6*, 63–94.

12. Giovanella, B.C., Stehlin, J.S., Shepard, R.C. and Williams, L.J. (1979): Hyperthermic treatment of human tumours heterotransplanted in nude mice. *Cancer Res., 39*, 2236–2241.

13. Hand, J.W. and Ter Haar, G. (1981): Heating techniques in hyperthermia. *Brit. J. Radiol., 54*, 443–446.

14. Har Kedar, I. and Bleehen, N.M. (1976): Experimental and clinical aspects of hyperthermia applied to the treatment of cancer. In: *Advances in Radiation Biology*, pp. 229–266. Editors: J.T. Lett and H. Adler. Academic Press, New York.

15. Herbst, H. and Sauer, R. (1980): First clinical results of local heating in combination with radiotherapy. In: *Proceedings, 1st Meeting of the European Group of Hyperthermia in Radiation Oncology*, pp. 267–275. Editors: G. Arcangeli and F. Mauro. Masson, Milan.

16. Kim, J.H. and Hahn, E.W. (1979): Clinical and biological studies of localised hyperthermia. *Cancer Res., 39*, 2258–2261.

17. Kremkau, F.W. (1979): Cancer therapy with ultrasound: a historical review. *J. clin. Ultrasound, 7*, 287–300.
18. Larkin, J.M. (1979): A clinical investigation of total body hyperthermia as cancer therapy. *Cancer Res., 39*, 2252–2254.
19. Le Veen, H.H., Wapnick, S., Piccone, V., Falk, G. and Ahmed, N. (1976): Tumour eradication by radiofrequency therapy. *J. Amer. med. Ass., 235*, 2198–2220.
20. Mantyla, M.J. (1970): Regional blood flow in human tumours. *Cancer Res., 39*, 2304–2306.
21. Marmor, J.B., Pounds, D., Postic, T.B. and Hahn, G.M. (1979): Treatment of superficial human neoplasms by local hyperthermia induced by ultrasound. *Cancer, 43*, 188–197.
22. Neumann, H., Engelhardt, R., Fabricius, H.A., Stahn, R. and Lohr, G.W. (1980): Clinical observations on tumour patients treated by whole body hyperthermia and cytostatic drugs: initial clinical results. In: *Proceedings, 1st Meeting of the European Group of Hyperthermia in Radiation Oncology,* pp. 201–207. Editors: G. Arcangeli and F. Mauro. Masson, Milan.
23. Parks, L.C., Munabeery, D., Smith, D.P. and Neely, W.A. (1981): Treatment of far advanced bronchogenic carcinoma by extracorporeally induced systemic hyperthermia. *J. thor. cardiovasc. Surg., 78*, 883–892.
24. Pettigrew, R.T., Galt, J.M., Ludgate, C.M. and Smith, A.N. (1974): Clinical effects of whole body hyperthermia in advanced malignancy. *Brit. med. J., 2*, 679–682.
25. Pomp, H. (1978): Clinical application of hyperthermia in gynaecological malignant tumours. In: *Cancer Therapy by Hyperthermia and Radiation,* pp. 326–327. Editors: C. Streffer, D. Van Beuningen, F. Dietzel, E. Rottinger, J.E. Robinson, E. Scherer, S. Seeber and D.R. Trott. Urban and Schwarzenberg, Baltimore–Munich.
26. *Proceedings, International Symposium on Cancer Therapy by Hyperthermia and Radiation,* pp. 305. American College of Radiology, Washington.
27. Proceedings, 3rd International Symposium: Cancer Therapy by Hyperthermia, Drugs and Radiation. *J. nat. Cancer Inst. Monogr., 60*, 1981.
28. Proceedings, 5th L.H. Gray Memorial Conference. *Brit. J. Cancer, Suppl.,* 1981, in press.
29. Short, J.G. and Turner, P.F. (1981): Physical hyperthermia and cancer therapy. *Proc. IEEE, 68*, 133–142.
30. Stehlin, J.S., Giovanella, B.C., De Ipolyi, P.D. and Anderson, R.F. (1979): Results of eleven years' experience with heated perfusion for melanoma of the extremities. *Cancer Res., 39*, 2255–2257.
31. Storm, F.K., Harrison, W.H., Elliott, R.S. and Morton, D.L. (1979): Normal tissue and solid tumour effects of hyperthermia in animal models and clinical trials. *Cancer Res., 39*, 2245–2251.
32. Warren, S.L. (1935): Preliminary study of the effect of artificial fever upon hopeless tumour cases. *Cancer, 33*, 75–87.

Recent progress in the pathology of lung neoplasms

B.F. Trump*, T. Wilson and C.C. Harris

Much progress has been made in recent years on the pathological diagnosis and clinicopathological correlations of bronchogenic carcinoma. This progress has resulted from at least 6 factors:

1. Application of electron-microscopic (EM) techniques to diagnosis and classification.
2. Increased use of cytochemistry including immunocytochemistry for characteristic markers.
3. Comparison of animal models with human neoplasms.
4. Studies of preneoplastic lesions and tumor promoters including wound repair in humans and experimental models.
5. Studies of animal and human bronchi in vitro including their response to carcinogens and putative promoters.
6. Comparison of cytological features of neoplasms and carcinogen metabolism with epidemiological data.

In the bronchus, as in other target organs in humans and experimental models, the development of neoplasia requires long periods of time during which successive populations of altered cells (preneoplastic lesions) occur prior to the appearance of invasive and metastatic neoplasms. These preneoplastic stages have altered cytoplasmic phenotypes as well as altered nuclear morphology.

The concept of initiation and promotion was formulated long ago. More recently, the mechanistic basis of this phenomenon is being clarified. At the present time, however, much more needs to be learned about tumor promotion in the tracheobronchial epithelium (TBE).

At the present time, little is known about the mechanisms involved in phenotypic differences in the final neoplasm, even in the same organ using the same carcinogen. Bronchogenic neoplasia is a good example. All students of the disease have been bewildered by the plethora of morphological phenotypes, often occurring simultaneously, making any attempt at classification very confusing. To some extent, these may relate to etiology, e.g. the high incidence of small-cell carcinomas in uranium miners or the adenocarcinoma of Chinese women in Hong Kong (20),

*The author is an 'American Cancer Society Professor of Clinical Oncology'.

but to a large extent such relationships are not understood. We are confronted, for example, by studies such as that of Vincent and colleagues (45) who commented on the changing histopathology of lung cancer; this group presented evidence that this is not due to changing criteria of diagnosis. The introduction of EM and cytochemical techniques to lung tumor diagnosis, however, has clearly improved our recognition of human phenotypes. Only the future can tell whether such improved classification will have an impact on lung cancer epidemiology and treatment.

PATHOLOGICAL FEATURES OF HUMAN BRONCHOGENIC CARCINOMA

We have recently proposed a phenotypic classification of lung carcinomas based on the phenotypic characteristics of the cytoplasm (5, 24) in over 150 human lung carcinomas. The carcinomas were a consecutive series, removed at surgery, and, therefore, represented a selected population (Table 1). Table 1 shows that a small number of tumors were bronchiolar and/or alveolar in origin; these will not be discussed. We have also studied tracheobronchial tumors of hamsters induced by intratracheal instillation of benzo(a)pyrene-ferric oxide (5). A comparison of our phenotypic classification of bronchogenic carcinomas with the 1967 World Health Organization Classification is shown in Table 2.

Cellular criteria of differentiation

Epidermoid carcinomas

Characteristic ultrastructural features include the presence of bundles of 100 mm tonofilaments, putatively keratin, and relatively poorly-developed endoplasmic reticulum and Golgi apparatus. In *well-differentiated tumors,* the tonofilaments are often seen to closely approach the cell membrane in the vicinity of the numerous prominent desmosomes. Lateral cell membranes are widely separated and commonly have long, well-formed microvilli and folds. The widened intercellular spaces are bridged by the apposing cell processes at the site of the desmosomes to form the so-called 'intercellular bridges' of light microscopy. The mitochondria are small and sparse. Various cell shapes are seen that range from polyhedral to spindle. Although keratohyalin granules are present in highly differentiated tumors, poorly differentiated tumors have relatively inconspicuous tonofilaments and desmosomes, and narrow intercellular spaces; intercellular bridges are not visible by light microscopy.

TABLE 1. *Phenotypic classification of lung carcinomas*

Tumor types	Percent based on 150 tumors*	
Characteristics of mucous and/or basal cells	87	
1. Epidermoid carcinoma	17	
Moderate to well-differentiated		13
Poorly differentiated		4
2. Combined epidermoid and adenocarcinoma	49	
A. Epidermoid component well-differentiated. 'Adeno' component well-differentiated		4
B. Epidermoid component well-differentiated. 'Adeno' component poorly differentiated		13
C. Epidermoid component poorly differentiated. 'Adeno' component well-differentiated		
I. Gross glandular organization		12
II. Solid pattern		12
D. Epidermoid component poorly differentiated. 'Adeno' component poorly differentiated		8
3. Adenocarcinoma	21	
I. Gross glandular organization		11
II. Solid pattern		10
Characteristics of endocrine cells	9	
1. Carcinoid	2	
2. Oat-cell	3	
3. Atypical	4	
Characteristics of Clara cells Adenocarcinoma Gross glandular organization	1.3	
Characteristics of Type II cells Adenocarcinoma Gross glandular organization	1.3	
Unclassified	1.3	

*These figures are derived from a consecutive surgical series. Therefore, the percent based on 150 tumors does not reflect the incidence of these tumors.

TABLE 2. *Comparison of histogenetic classification with WHO classification*

Study	WHO	
Tumors with characteristics of mucous and/or basal cells		
1. Epidermoid carcinoma		
Well-differentiated	Epidermoid	I
Moderately differentiated	Combined epidermoid and adenocarcinoma*	V
Poorly differentiated		
Small-cell type	Small-cell anaplastic	II
Large-cell type	Large-cell solid	IV
2. Combined epidermoid and adenocarcinoma		
A. Epidermoid component, well-differentiated.	Combined epidermoid and adenocarcinoma	V
'Adeno' component, well-differentiated		
B. Epidermoid component, well-differentiated.	Epidermoid	I
'Adeno' component, poorly differentiated	Combined epidermoid and adenocarcinoma*	V
C. Epidermoid component, poorly differentiated.		
'Adeno' component, well-differentiated		
I. Gross structural organization maintained	Adenocarcinoma	III
II. Gross structural organization lost	Large-cell solid	IV
D. Epidermoid component, poorly differentiated.	Small-cell anaplastic	II
'Adeno' component, poorly differentiated	Large-cell solid	IV
3. Adenocarcinoma		
I. Gross structural organization maintained	Adenocarcinoma	III
II. Gross structural organization lost	Large-cell solid	IV
Tumors with characteristics of endocrine cells		
1. Carcinoid	Carcinoid	VI
2. Oat-cell carcinoma	Small-cell anaplastic 'Oat-cell'	II
3. Atypical	Large-cell solid	IV

*Ducts lined by non-neoplastic cells may be trapped in epidermoid cell nests, giving the erroneous impression of combined epidermoid and adenocarcinomas (24).

Adenocarcinomas

Characteristic ultrastructural features are those associated with cell secretion. These include an extensive rough endoplasmic reticulum, a large Golgi apparatus and numerous mitochondria. The cells are joined by desmosomes, but these are relatively poorly-developed. Typical junctional complexes may also be present at the luminal aspect of cells when several cells form an acinus surrounding an extracellular alveolus. However, extracellular alveoli may be absent and only intracellular alveoli are present. These small alveoli commonly contain flocculent material which stains for mucosubstances. Discrete secretory granules, such as mucous or putative endocrine granules (dense-core granules), may also be seen. Therefore, the diagnosis of adenocarcinoma is based on the presence of one or more of the following criteria: the presence of extra- and/or intracellular alveoli; well-developed Golgi apparatus; and endoplasmic reticulum and/or other evidence of cellular secretion.

Tumors with characteristics of mucous and/or basal cells

Eighty-seven percent of the tumors fell into this group (Table 1). The tumors were subdivided into epidermoid carcinomas, combined epidermoid and adenocarcinomas, and adenocarcinomas, as described below.

Epidermoid carcinomas

Seventeen percent of carcinomas were of this type (Table 1). The tumor cells have some characteristics of normal basal cells even in poorly differentiated tumors. The epidermoid characteristics of well-differentiated and poorly differentiated carcinomas are described above (cellular criteria of differentiation). We are of the opinion that epidermoid carcinomas, presenting various degrees of differentiation, have been previously classified as Groups I, II, IV and V using the WHO classification (Table 2).

Combined epidermoid and adenocarcinomas

Forty-nine percent of carcinomas were placed in this large group (Table 1). The tumors have cytoplasmic features of both basal and mucous cells. The epidermoid and 'adeno' components of combined tumors are recognized by the cellular criteria of differentiation as described above. Combined epidermoid and adenocarcinomas have been previously classified as Groups I, II, III, IV and V using the WHO classification (Table 2).

Combined epidermoid and adenocarcinomas exhibit a broad spectrum of differentiation (Tables 1 and 2). Tumors range from those where both components are quantitatively well-represented and neither component appears to be dominant, to tumors where one component is quite clearly dominant over the other. However, the classification of combined tumors is dependent not only upon the relative amounts of the different differentiation patterns but also upon the degree of differentiation of each component.

Epidermoid component, well-differentiated; 'adeno' component, well-differentiated
In H&E-stained sections, these tumors are composed of nests of polygonal cells, often showing keratinization and joined by intercellular bridges. However, numerous extracellular alveoli lie within the epidermoid cell nests; these alveoli are often filled with mucus. Intracellular mucus-filled alveoli are also seen in some cells. Ultrastructural examination reveals features characteristic of well-differentiated epidermoid carcinomas. However, junctional complexes join the cells together where the apposed cell membranes border the glandular lumens, forming extracellular alveoli; mucous secretion is abundant.

Epidermoid component, well-differentiated; 'adeno' component, poorly differentiated
In H&E sections, the tumors appear as well- or moderately well-differentiated epidermoid carcinomas. However, histochemical stains reveal mucus in intra- and extracellular alveoli, but these are not widespread. In individual cells of some tumors, mucous granules are seen in the cytoplasm. At the ultrastructural level, most of the cells are typically epidermoid, but focal areas of adenocarcinoma differentiation are seen.

Epidermoid component, poorly differentiated; 'adeno' component, well-differentiated
Keratinization and intercellular bridges are not recognizable by light microscopy, but the epidermoid component is represented ultrastructurally by well-developed desmosomes and by the presence of tonofilament bundles which may be plentiful or sparse. The endoplasmic reticulum and Golgi apparatus tend to be well-developed and the tumors usually secrete copious amounts of mucus. These tumors fall into two subgroups depending upon their gross glandular organization:
Gross glandular organization maintained – Subgroup I Using the WHO criteria, tumors of this type would be classified as Group III adenocarcinomas (Table 2). Gross glandular organization is maintained and the cells are joined at the luminal surface by junctional complexes

and laterally by desmosomes. Tonofilament bundles are present in the cells in varying amounts. Histochemical stains often demonstrate mucus, not only within the glandular lumens, but also in intracellular alveoli, which appear as punctate droplets by light microscopy.

Gross glandular organization minimal – Subgroup II Gross glandular organization is minimal and the tumors largely assume a solid growth pattern. Tumors of this type would be classified as Group IV, large-cell carcinoma, using the WHO criteria (Table 2). The morphology of the cells which comprise the neoplasm is very similar to that described above in Subgroup I. Intracellular and small extracellular alveoli are abundant and mucus-filled. The cells are joined by numerous desmosomes and bundles of tonofilaments are present. Junctional complexes join the apices of cells where the cells abut small extracellular alveoli. Endoplasmic reticulum and Golgi apparatus are well-developed and multivesicular bodies are often present.

Epidermoid component, poorly differentiated; 'adeno' component, poorly differentiated
Keratinization and/or intercellular bridging is not evident at light-microscopic level; depending on cell size and shape, these tumors would certainly be placed in Groups II (small cells) and IV (large cells) of the WHO classification (Table 2). In rare focal areas, mucus-filled alveoli are present and in the apices of the cells which form the alveoli, tiny mucous droplets can be seen.

At the ultrastructural level, the cell borders are seen to be closely apposed, yet desmosomes and tonofilament bundles are present. The endoplasmic reticulum is quite well-developed in some tumors of this type.

Summary and synthesis: combined epidermoid and adenocarcinomas
Combined epidermoid and adenocarcinomas have generally been considered rare tumors (18). According to the WHO classification, the diagnosis of these tumors is dependent upon the presence of tubules and gland-like structures, as well as areas that exhibit epidermoid differentiation. However, when the phenotypic criteria for epidermoid and adenocarcinoma differentiation are used in the classification of lung carcinomas, combined tumors are found to be very common. Some light-microscopic studies have recognized combined epidermoid and adenocarcinomas as a significant entity (36), but other investigators have commented on pseudogland formation in epidermoid carcinomas (33) or have described focal areas of squamous metaplasia in adenocarcinomas (36). Walter and Pryce (45) noted that in 2 cases of primary epidermoid carcinomas, the secondary metastases were adenocarcinomas.

Increased use of the electron microscope in tumor diagnosis will undoubtedly increase the pathologist's awareness of the frequency of these combined tumors. The frequency of combined epidermoid and adenocarcinomas hardly seems surprising in light of our studies on regeneration and on the histogenesis of epidermoid metaplasia and carcinoma in situ in both human and hamster respiratory epithelium. We conclude that combined epidermoid-adenocarcinomas arise from columnar mucus-secreting epithelia, either from transformed mucous cells and/or transformed basal cells, which show differentiation for mucus production.

Adenocarcinomas

Neoplasms which fall in this category are morphologically similar to combined epidermoid and adenocarcinomas, where the epidermoid component is poorly differentiated and the 'adeno' component is well-differentiated (described above). However, the cells have minimal epidermoid differentiation: i.e., tonofilament bundles are scant and desmosomes are small. Depending on the gross organization of the tumor, the tumors fall into two subgroups:

Gross glandular organization maintained – Subgroup I
Such tumors would be classified as Group III adenocarcinomas, using the WHO criteria (Table 2). Adenocarcinomas which maintain gross glandular organization may or may not be mucus-producing.

Gross glandular organization minimal – Subgroup II
These tumors would be classified as Group IV, using the WHO classification (Table 2). The tumor cells are seen growing in solid masses and may or may not secret mucus. Often a few focal areas of tubular formation are retained in an otherwise solid tumor. Extracellular alveoli may appear slit-like, so that they are not immediately recognizable by light microscopy, except by the use of mucous stains. The endoplasmic reticulum and Golgi apparatus are well developed. Intracellular alveoli and small slit-like extracellular alveoli are easily recognized ultrastructurally; desmosomes are small and tonofilament bundles inconspicuous.

Histogenesis and environmental factors

In our ongoing study of carcinomas, 87% of the tumors had characteristics of basal and/or mucous cells. Tumors included in this group were epidermoid carcinomas, combined epidermoid and adenocarcinomas, and adenocarcinomas. Of all the tumors in this large group, 66% of the tumors showed varying degrees of epidermoid differentiation, while 21% of the tumors showed virtually none (Table 1).

As discussed below, our recent data (5, 42) clearly suggest that epidermoid metaplasia and carcinoma in situ can arise from modulations of mucous cells. These cells show varying degrees of epidermoid differentiation. Epidermoid metaplasia also occurs in regenerating epithelium in the absence of carcinogenic stimulation (23). Could these modulations of differentiation be purely under environmental control? It is well known that certain differentiation patterns are subject to modulation by the microenvironment. For example, epithelia of the urogenital and respiratory tracts undergo epidermoid metaplasia in vivo in vitamin-A-deficient states (50); similar changes can be induced in vitro. For example, prostatic epithelium (19) and respiratory epithelium (10) become keratinized when cultured in vitamin-A-deficient media, whereas mucus secretion is maintained in complete medium. Conversely, non-mucus-secreting epithelia become mucus-secreting in vitro upon addition of excess vitamin A (51). Furthermore, topical application of vitamin A to keratoacanthomas induces mucous metaplasia in the tumors (29) and addition of retinoids to prostate gland in explant culture reverses hyperplastic lesions induced by chemical carcinogens (9). Additionally, Yuspa and colleagues (52) have shown that extracellular calcium can modify keratin operation and controlled epithelium.

Some experiments have investigated the roles of both cellular and environmental factors. The formation of cysts and junctional complexes ('adeno' features) were found to be responses to a liquid environment when cervical squamous carcinoma cell-lines were grown in vitro (2). In a study of a bladder cell-line, confluent horizontal monolayers became piled up and stratified, and aggregated at the aerobic end of the gradient when the culture tubes were placed vertically; in addition, the cells became keratinized (41).

Thus, it appears that features of differentiation are subject to modulation by the microenvironment. These data further indicate that factors other than the cell of origin can influence differentiation patterns exhibited by tumors. Since environmental influences may vary, so different types of phenotypic expression may vary in the same tumor, despite a common histogenetic origin.

Tumors with putative endocrine cells

As discussed above, current concepts on the histogenesis of carcinoid tumors and oat-cell carcinomas stem from the premise that presumptive endocrine cells of the bronchial epithelium are the cells of origin of these tumors. We have presented evidence which suggests that this may not always be the case.

The epithelial lining of the respiratory tract is of endodermal origin.

Bronchial buds are originally lined by a simple epithelium which later differentiates into one that is pseudostratified. Basal cells, mucous cells and ciliated cells presumably derive from this simple epithelium, whereas the origin of endocrine cells in respiratory epithelium is less well-established. One hypothesis was that endocrine cells were derived, not from entoderm, but from cells of the neural crest (28). However, sufficient evidence now exists to suggest that endocrine cells of the gastro-enteropancreatic system do not arise from the neural crest (34). A possible interpretation is that, in some way, cells of common endodermal origin are programmed in early fetal development to differentiate into basal, mucous, ciliated or endocrine cells, perhaps influenced by microenvironmental factors.

In normal gastrointestinal epithelium, transitional forms between argentaffin cells and mucous cells were described using light-microscopic histochemistry (32) and electron microscopy (8); presumptive endocrine granules were observed at ultrastructural level in mucous cells of normal human bronchi (40). In this regard, Tateishi (39) remarked upon the fact that argyrophilic cells (presumptively endocrine cells) in human bronchi and bronchioles were often found closely associated with areas of mucous goblet-cell hyperplasia.

These observations made on non-neoplastic epithelia, together with descriptions of the presence of mucosubstances and presumptive endocrine granules in tumors of endodermal origin (reviewed in Ref. 34), provide evidence against the neuroectodermal origin of the endocrine cells in endodermally derived epithelia.

Carcinoid tumors

Detailed reports with regard to the histogenesis of carcinoid tumors are those of Hage (13) and Capella and colleagues (7). Hage (13) described the ultrastructural morphology of 6 bronchial carcinoid tumors. The individual tumors were composed of 1, 2 or even 3 apparently different types of endocrine cells, based on the morphological and cytochemical characteristics of the granules. Two of the 3 cell types found in the tumors appeared similar to endocrine cells normally found in the respiratory epithelium of human fetuses. In contrast, in the study of Capella and colleagues (7), 2 distinct tumor types were described. One tumor type was composed entirely of small granule cells, the other type of large granule cells; small and large granule cells were not observed in single tumors.

The unusual carcinoid tumor described by McDowell and colleagues (25) and Sorokin and colleagues (35) was unusual, in that it presented with a spectrum of granule morphologies and cells of the tumor had as many as 10 different cytochemical staining signatures. The relationships of this tumor to the intraepithelial clusters of abnormal endocrine cells have been described above. The tumor was composed of polygonal cells, some of which had long cytoplasmic processes. The plasma membranes closely paralleled each other, so that intercellular spaces were minimal. The cytoplasm contained round to elongate mitonchondria, a prominent Golgi complex, some stacks of rough endoplasmic reticulum and free ribosomes. Residual bodies containing lipofuscin were commonly observed.

Small-cell anaplastic carcinomas, including oat-cell carcinomas

Small-cell anaplastic carcinomas present a variety of histological patterns. The tumors appear very cellular and the nuclear to cytoplasmic ratio is high. Subtypes include the lymphocyte or oat-cell type and polygonal and fusiform variants (8).

Whereas some small-cell anaplastic carcinomas are composed of small cells showing poorly differentiated features of epidermoid and/or mucus-secreting adenocarcinoma differentiation (24), many tumors, including the oat-cell variety, are composed of cells which exhibit endocrine differentiation (Table 2).

Typically, oat-cell tumors of the lung are characterized by the small oat-shaped cells, which resemble lymphocytes but which may be up to twice the size of lymphocytes. The small cells, with a very high nuclear to cytoplasmic ratio, may be seen arranged in streams, ribbons, rosettes, tubules or ductules (3). Dense-core secretory granules ranging from 800 Å to 2000 Å in diameter are present within the cytoplasm, especially concentrated in cytoplasmic processes (6, 15).

Less widely recognized, although it has been known for many years, is the fact that foci of tubular differentiation and/or foci of epidermoid (squamous) differentiation may be present in small-cell anaplastic carcinomas of the lung. In an early description of pulmonary oat-cell carcinoma (oat-cell sarcoma), Barnard (4) described spindle and polygonal cells of intermediate size, intermingled among the characteristic small 'oat' cells. In some of these tumors, the oat-cells were focally aligned to form small tubules. Walter and Pryce (45) described tubules and rosettes (poorly formed tubules) in 48% of oat-cell tumors; however, staining for mucus was negative. They also described foci of squamous metaplasia in some of these tumors. The tubules were filled with mucosubstances that were PAS- and mucicarmine-positive. These substances also stained weakly with Alcian blue. Intracellular mucosubstances were not reported. Willis (48) and Lisa and colleagues (21) reported that tubule and duct formation occurred frequently in oat-cell carcinomas, although mucus was seen only infrequently; 'squamoid cells' were also seen. Watson and Berg (47) described keratinization in an oat-cell carcinoma and Koss (17) considered oat-cell carcinomas to be poorly differentiated epidermoid carcinomas of small-cell type, because of foci of epidermoid differentiation. Koss (17) also noted a tendency towards glandular formation in some of these tumors.

We have recently described a tumor with presumptive endocrine granules, mucous secretion and tonofilament bundles (keratin, unpublished observations), in the same cells (26). The tumor was composed of small cells containing argyrophilic dense-core granules. Foci of epidermoid differentiation and foci of glandular differentiation associated with intra- and extracellular secretion of acidic mucosubstances were also seen. In some areas, glandular mucus-filled hollows were surrounded by cells which were joined apically by junctional complexes and laterally by very large, well-developed desmosomes. These cells contained large and numerous tonofilament bundles as well as two morphologically distinct types of granules: dense-core endocrine-type granules and mucous granules. The tumor clearly arose from terminal bronchi and foci of basally situated hyperplastic and/or neoplastic cells were seen beneath otherwise normal columnar-ciliated epithelium.

Atypical endocrine tumors

Due to increasing use of the electron microscope in tumor diagnosis in recent years, sporadic reports have described neurosecretory granules, dense-core granules, 'carcinoid-like' granules or 'inclusion bodies' in a few primary lung tumors which demonstrated neither carcinoid nor oat-cell characteristics on light-microscopic examination. These tumors were classified as anaplastic carcinomas (38), adenocarcinomas (14) or as large-cell carcinomas (14). Although all of these studies reported upon the presence of endocrine-type cytoplasmic dense-core granules, only Gould and Chejfec (12) attempted to elucidate the chemical component(s) of the granules. They were able to demonstrate 5-hydroxy-3-indoleacetic acid, vanillylmandelic acid and catecholamine activity associated with two large-cell 'undifferentiated' carcinomas which contained dense-core granules.

During the course of examining the 150 lung tumors by light and electron microscopy, we found that 7 malignant peripheral lung tumors, which were diagnosed by 3 different pathologists by routine light microscopy either as epidermoid and/or adenocarcinomas (showing varying degrees of differentiation) or as large-cell carcinomas, also contained characteristic dense-core putative endocrine granules (27). By light microscopy, the tumors were composed of nests of large cells.

Often these nests had necrotic centers. The nuclei were anaplastic, nucleoli were large and prominent, and mitotic figures were frequent. Four of the 7 tumors were mucus-producing. The cells were joined by desmosomes and contained well-developed bundles of tonofilaments (keratin, unpublished observations). Using the peroxidase antiperoxidase method, serotonin-positive cells were demonstrated in 6 of the 7 tumors and argyrophilic granules were demonstrated at the ultrastructural level in 5 of 6 tumors tested (see also below). All tumors extended to the visceral pleura and two invaded both pleural layers, with extension to the chest wall at the time of surgery. None of the tumors was classified as carcinoid, small-cell anaplastic or oat-cell tumors, even in focal areas, by any of the pathologists. Thus, for want of a better descriptive name, we have called these tumors 'atypical endocrine tumors' (27).

Summary and synthesis

We have described argyrophilic presumptive endocrine granules in cells bearing cilia or mucous granules in the bronchial epithelium associated with a pulmonary carcinoid tumor and we have described tripartite differentiation, i.e. presumptive endocrine granules, mucous granules and keratin filaments, within single cells of a small-cell anaplastic carcinoma. Dense-core granules and mucous granules have also been described within the same cells of goblet-cell carcinoid tumors of the appendix (1, 47). Recently, Ewing and colleagues (11) have reported on 437 cases of pulmonary small-cell anaplastic carcinoma. Fourteen tumors showed, in addition to the small-cell component, areas of differentiation into another cell type. Combinations of small cell–epidermoid, small cell–'adeno', small–combined epidermoid and 'adeno', and small cell–large cell undifferentiated carcinoma were described. The specimens showing mixed histological patterns were obtained prior to radiation or chemotherapy. The finding of an additional group of tumors – atypical endocrine tumors of the lung – with multiple patterns of differentiation, i.e. putative endocrine dense-core granules together with epidermoid differentiation (well-developed tonofilament bundles and desmosomes) and foci of glandular differentiation associated with intra- and extracellular secretion of mucosubstances, gives further support to our ideas relating to the histogenesis of lung tumors with endocrine differentiation. We believe that these tumors, including carcinoid and oat-cell tumors, may not necessarily derive from malignant transformation of respiratory endocrine cells, as proposed by current dogma. Instead, we believe that tumors with an endocrine phenotype may sometimes arise from non-endocrine cells within the epithelium which have been driven by carcinogenic stimuli towards expressing an endocrine cell phenotype. To what extent the affected cells are drawn from hypothetical stem cells, from a pool of pre-existing endocrine cells, or from indifferent cells derived by division of non-endocrine cells, i.e. basal and/or mucous cells, remains unknown (37).

CYTOPATHOLOGICAL DIAGNOSIS

The increasing importance of this technique in analysis of sputum, bronchial washings and aspiration needle biopsies requires that this method be given increasing scrutiny. There have been several recent studies comparing analysis with this technique with the diagnosis made histopathology. Studies in our laboratory indicate that much better correlations exist when newer criteria, developed on the basis of ultrastructure and cytochemistry, are used to classify the histopathology. Because of the increased resolution of cytological detail, the cytopathological technique may give a better idea of the ultrastructural differentiation than the use of H&E or special stains on paraffin sections (16).

In the future, the application of immunocytochemical markers to cytopathology may yield many further improvements.

IMMUNOCYTOCHEMICAL MARKERS

On the basis of the qualitative and quantitative results of our immunohistochemical studies, the histological range of human lung cancer appears to be divisible into 4 broad groups (Table 3). These are: (1) tumors with a well-differentiated epidermoid component of differentiation, regardless of adenocarcinomatous differentiation, (2) tumors of poorly differentiated epidermoid differentiation, with or without adenocarcinomatous differentiation or adenocarcinomas without epidermoid differentiation, (3) Clara cell adenocarcinomas, and (4) endocrine tumors. These groups correspond to the histogenetic tumor types described by McDowell and colleagues (22, 27) as follows: (1) well-differentiated epidermoid carcinoma, CEAC/A, CEAC/B; (2) poorly differentiated epidermoid carcinoma, CEAC/CI, CEAC/CII, CEAC/D, ACI, ACII; (3) CAC; and (4) atypical endocrine tumors, carcinoids and small-cell carcinomas.

Group 1 tumors were characterized by (a) keratin immunoreactivity in nearly all cells which varied from cell to cell in intensity, (b) somatostatin (60%) and CEA (95%) reactivity in large cells at the center keratinizing nests. These tumors lacked serotonin and neuron-specific enolase (NSE), and rarely contained α-fetoprotein and calcitonin. ACTH was observed in 57%, but was variably distributed. HCG-B was

TABLE 3. *Immunohistochemical marker distribution as a function of histogenetic tumor type*

	ACT4		α-Fetoprotein		Calcitonin		CEA		HCG-B		Keratin		NSE		Serotonin	
	n	%+	n	%+	n	%+	n	%+	n	%+	n	%+	n	%+	n	%+
wdEC	10	50	10	0	10	0	7	100	10	100	10	100	2	0	10	0
pdEC	10	50	10	0	10	20	9	44	10	80	10	90	2	0	10	0
CEAC/A	10	80	10	10	10	20	3	100	10	100	10	100	2	0	10	0
CEAC/B	10	40	10	0	10	0	8	88	10	100	10	100	2	0	10	0
CEAC/CI	10	40	10	0	10	20	5	100	10	80	10	80	2	0	10	0
CEAC/CII	10	60	10	10	10	50	7	86	10	90	10	80	2	0	10	0
CEAC/D	10	20	10	0	10	10	7	57	10	70	10	70	2	0	10	0
ACI	9	95	9	11	9	11	10	100	9	100	9	67	2	0	9	0
ACII	10	30	10	0	10	10	6	67	10	80	10	60	2	0	10	0
CAC	4	25	4	0	4	75	1	100	4	100	4	50	4	0	4	0
Atypical endocrine	7	43	7	0	7	29	0	-	7	100	7	100	7	100	7	88
Carcinoid	2	50	2	0	2	50	6	100	2	50	2	0	2	100	2	50
SCC	10	0	10	0	10	0	3	100	10	0	10	20	10	100	10	0

n = number of tumors stained; %+ = % of stained tumors with immunoreactivity of any degree. For further explanation, see text.

present in 100% of these tumors, generally following the distribution of glycogen, but this finding was typical of Group 2 and Group 3 tumors, as well as of the atypical endocrine tumors of Group 4 (49).

Group 2 tumors were characterized by: (a) a slightly lower proportion of keratin-reactive tumors, and a weaker and more uniform keratin pattern than tumors of Group 1; (b) a generally similar proportion of CEA-reactive tumors, in which reactivity tended toward intra- and extracellular luminal surfaces; (c) a slightly lower proportion of ACTH- and somatostatin-reactive tumors, in which reactivity tended to be more diffuse than in Group 1; (d) a slightly larger proportion of calcitonin-reactive tumors, with more diffuse staining than in Group 1. These tumors also lacked serotonin and NSE.

Group 3 tumors were characterized by a relatively low (50%) incidence of keratin and a relatively high (75%) calcitonin incidence as compared to Groups 1 and 2. CEA was present intracellularly. These tumors also lacked α-fetoprotein, somatostatin, NSE and serotonin. These results may be colored by a rather small (n = 4) sample size.

Group 4 tumors were placed together on the morphological basis that they all contained endocrine granules, and on the histochemical basis that they all contained NSE and that they are the only group which included tumors positive for NSE and serotonin. In other respects, they were composed of 3 histochemically distinct tumor types. The atypical endocrine tumors were highly reactive for most markers, including keratin, HCG-B, NSE, serotonin, somatostatin and, to a lesser degree, ACTH and calcitonin. Carcinoids, again a small sample (n = 2), included one highly reactive tumor and one generally unreactive tumor, and represented an immunohistochemical middle ground between the highly reactive atypical endocrine tumors and the virtually unreactive small-cell tumors. Carcinoids and small-cell carcinomas reacted for CEA intracellularly or at the cell borders.

PRENEOPLASTIC LESIONS AND HISTOGENESIS

According to current concepts, carcinogenesis is a multistage process beginning with the initiated cell and terminating with invasive, metastasizing cancer. It appears from both human and animal data that the early stages are potentially reversible. Indeed, the early stages may be indistinguishable following carcinogenic or non-carcinogenic injuries.

In the bronchus in both human and experimental neoplasia, the following stages are commonly recognized: epidermoid ('squamous') metaplasia with progressive nuclear atypia: dysplasia with progressive nuclear atypia: carcinoma in situ; and invasive carcinoma. These

116

changes appear sequentially in both animals and man, although it should be understood that, since the lesions are typically multiple, the changes of the most advanced stage are usually mixed with cells showing less advanced stages in a sputum cytological specimen.

Although the first commonly recognized lesion is epidermoid metaplasia, such lesions are commonly mixed with mucous-cell hyperplasia, a common early reaction to injury. All of these early lesions are probably related to the sequence of changes seen in epithelial wound repair (see below).

Acute injury and repair sequence

Several studies have been performed in which the tracheal epithelium in rodents is injured by scraping away the epithelial cells down to the basal lamina in a given site in the trachea and then following the sequence of repair and reconstitution. The most detailed such experiments have been carried out by McDowell and colleagues (23). Within 2 hours after scraping, virtually all cells had sloughed from the injured area, leaving a virtually bare basal lamina. Between 6 and 12 hours, the adjacent basal and mucous cells flatten, becoming squamous, and migrate from the margins, partially covering the denuded basal lamina. Increased cell division was not noted at these times. Many of the squamous cells resembled mucous cells with well-developed endoplasmic reticulum and Golgi apparatus and mucus, while others resembled basal cells. By 24 hours, the defect was covered by one or two layers of squamous cells and at this time many were in division; cell division was also increased in both mucous and basal cells in the uninjured epithelium distant from the defect. By 48 hours in the area of the wound, the epithelium was stratified and contained cells that were typical of epidermoid metaplasia, comprising several layers of polygonal or flattened cells containing abundant keratin filaments and also stainable mucosubstances. By 72 hours, large numbers of so-called indifferent cells were seen extending to the luminal surface. These seem to have been derived, at least in part, from division of the metaplastic mucus-producing cells. These indifferent cells then differentiate into ciliated cells often through a ciliated mucous form, apparently recapitulating differentiation as it occurs in the primitive, undifferentiated epithelium of the fetal airway (23). Indifferent cells should not be confused with basal cells or so-called 'reserve cells'. These cells are tall cuboidal to columnar with pale cytoplasm and appear to arise from division of any cell in the normal epithelium which retains the capacity to divide, i.e. basal cells, mucous cells and possibly endocrine cells.

At present, little is known concerning the factors which modify differentiation and/or phenotypic expressions. Retinoids can evidently influence differentiation toward mucous secretion and retinoid deficiency toward epidermal metaplasia. The mechanism of both these is unknown, but important to characterize if more than empirical therapy is desired. The fact, however, that intracellular calcium can influence the development of keratin and since retinoids are known to modify cellular membranes, it may be that keratin differentiation reflects an abnormality of intracellular ionized calcium. There is also evidence that certain carcinogens favor the genesis of one type of neoplasm over another, which may again be the result of modulation by microenvironmental factors. Nitrosamines, for example, seem to favor proliferations of cells containing endocrine-like granules in the hamster, whereas benzo(a)pyrene with ferric oxide seems to result in the genesis of epidermoid carcinomas and mucus-secreting combined epidermoid adenocarcinomas.

Acute ischemic injury

In our studies of acute ischemic injury in the hamster trachea and the human bronchus, the reactions to total ischemia in vitro resemble those seen in many other organs, although the time scale of progression is somewhat slower. Hamster tracheal epithelium can survive 3 hours of total ischemia at 37 °C and much longer at reduced temperatures. By 3 hours of ischemia, which is reversible in the hamster, the cells are markedly altered. The mucous cells show increased densifications of the cytoplasm, swelling of mitochondria and endoplasmic reticulum, and distortion of the microvilli. The ciliated cells are also dramatically altered, again with cytoplasmic and mitochondrial swelling and the frequent presence of large blebs at the surface incorporating several ciliary axonemes. The latter change resembles that seen after treatment of these cells with a calcium ionophore (31); as we reviewed recently, these rapid shape-changes probably reflect the effects of increased cytosol-ionized calcium on the cytoskeleton, including both contractile filaments and microtubules (43). Whether or not actual deciliation of such cells might occur is unknown. It is clear that lowering of extracellular calcium in some ciliated cells can result in a somewhat similar process, with removal of cilia and re-entry of the cells into the mitotic cycle.

Goblet cell 'hyperplasia'

Increased numbers and size of 'goblet cells' or other cells containing mucous granules is a commonly observed reaction to either carcinogenic or non-carcinogenic stimuli such as the reaction known as bronchitis.

118

Although it is intimately related to epidermoid metaplasia as mentioned below, it appears to be an earlier stage, although in many human cases or after experimental treatment with carcinogens, both goblet-cell hyperplasia and epidermoid metaplasia coexist and abrupt transitions from one to the other are commonly seen. In experimental injuries, early after irritation there is loss of ciliated cells by extrusion and mitotic figures are occasionally observed in luminal small mucous granule cells. Distention of cells with mucous granules in large continuous areas virtually free of ciliated cells can be commonly observed. The exact mechanism resulting in the accumulation of mucus is not clear, but it is clear that mucous cells can divide and that ciliated cells are easily extruded following injury resulting in this form.

Epidermoid metaplasia

In epidermoid metaplasia in both humans and experimental animals, the changes blend into goblet-cell hyperplasia. It appears that later after stimulation the mucous cells begin to pile up or stratify and most of the large mucous granules are lost or secreted. It is easy, however, to detect numerous mucous granules within all of the stratified layers except the basal layer itself. At this point, however, in addition to the phenotypic changes, some of the cells produce much more keratin. It is our hypothesis that the stimulus for the epidermoid metaplasia is that the more severe injury results in modulation of intracellular calcium which sets the stage for keratin filament production. The type of mucus that is produced becomes more sulfated and in epidermoid metaplasia the total amount decreases per cell. This might tend to perpetuate the injury as, at least in some cells, the secretion of glycosaminoglycans has been suggested to have an important defense role, its modification of the epithelial barrier minimizing external injurious influences.

Epidermoid metaplasia is also closely related to goblet-cell hyperplasia, from the histogenetic point of view. Both may result from carcinogens and presumably non-carcinogenic chemical irritants. Many studies indicate that both occur when the bronchus is exposed to irritants and, indeed, epidermoid metaplasia is often or usually preceded by mucous hyperplasia. In other experiments, goblet-cell hyperplasia was induced with low doses of cigarette smoke, while higher doses produced epidermoid metaplasia. The same occurred in our experiments with benzpyrene-treated hamster tracheas.

Hyperplasia of small granule cells

In experiments with nitrosamines, Reznik-Schuller (30) noted prolifera-

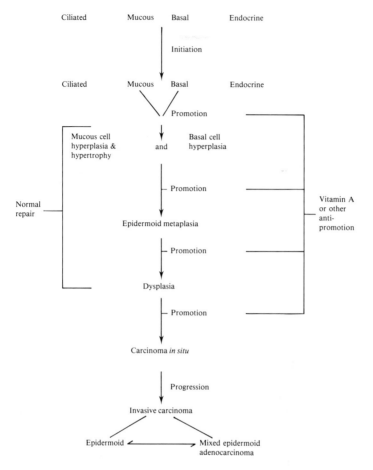

Fig. 1. *Present concept of tumor initiation, promotion, and progression in the bronchial epithelium.*

tion of 'endocrine'-type cells early in diethylnitrosamine-induced lung carcinogenesis. Recently, we have observed, in a case of a rather unusual carcinoid tumor, clusters of normal endocrine cells situated at the basal aspect of otherwise normal bronchial and bronchial-glandular epithelium. Some mucous cells and some ciliated cells were also noted within these clusters containing putative endocrine granules. Some of these clusters were isolated from one another as shown by serial sections. These clusters, therefore, represented hyperplastic, metaplastic and/or areas of carcinoma in situ composed of normal endocrine cells, some of which had mixed endocrine and non-endocrine phenotypes.

120

SUMMARY

Figure 1 gives a summary of our present concept of tumor initiation, promotion and progression in the bronchial epithelium. The example given is for epidermoid or mixed epidermoid-adenocarcinoma. Note that the types of preneoplastic lesions described above are visualized as the result of promotion; that they also can represent a part of these two types of neoplasms from mucous and/or basal cells is compatible with their mixed and probably unstable phenotype. The extent to which this instability is genetic versus microenvironmental cannot be presently determined. Also illustrated in the diagram are anti-promotion agents which may be able to inhibit carcinogenesis or even reverse preneoplastic stages. In the case of human bronchial carcinogenesis, the principal candidate is vitamin A and related retinoids.

References

1. Abt, A.B. and Carter, S.L. (1976): Goblet cell carcinoid of the appendix. *Arch. Path. Lab. Med., 100,* 301–306.
2. Auersperg, N. (1969): Histogenetic behavior of tumors. II. Roles of cellular and environmental factors in the in vitro growth of carcinoma cells. *J. nat. Cancer Inst., 43,* 175–190.
3. Azzopardi, J.G. (1959): Oat-cell carcinoma of the bronchus. *J. Path. Bact., 78,* 513–519.
4. Barnard, W.G. (1926): The nature of the 'oat-celled sarcoma' of the mediastinum. *J. Path. Bact., 29,* 241–244.
5. Becci, P.J., McDowell, E.M. and Trump, B.F. (1978): The respiratory epithelium. II. Hamster trachea, bronchus and bronchioles. *J. nat. Cancer Inst., 61,* 551–561.
6. Bensch, K.G., Corrin, B.J., Pariente, R. and Spencer, H. (1968): Oat cell carcinoma of the lung: its origin and relationship to bronchial carcinoid. *Cancer, 22,* 1163–1172.
7. Capella, C., Gabrielli, M., Polak, J.M., Buffa, R., Solcia, E. and Bordi, C. (1979): Ultrastructural and histological study of 11 bronchial carcinoids: evidence for different types. *Virchows Arch. Abt. A. Path. Anat., 381,* 313–329.
8. Chang, C. and Leblond, C.P. (1974): Origin, differentiation and renewal of the four main epithelial cell types in the mouse small intestine. V. Unitarian theory of the origin of the four epithelial cell types. *Amer. J. Anat., 141,* 537–548.
9. Chopra, D.P. and Wilkoff, L.J. (1976): Inhibition and reversal by α-retinoic acid of hyperplasia induced in cultured mouse prostate tissue by 3-methylcholanthrene or N-methyl-N'-nitrosoguanidine. *J. nat. Cancer Inst., 56,* 583–589.

10. Calmon, G.H., Spron, M.B., Smith, J.M. and Shaffiotti, U. (1974): α- and β-retinyl acetate reverses metaplasias of vitamin A deficiency in hamster trachea in organ culture. *Nature (Lond.), 250,* 64–66.

11. Ewing, S.L., Sumner, H.W., Ophoven, J.J., Mayer, J.E.J. and Humphrey, E.W. (1980): Small cell anaplastic carcinoma with differentiation: a report of 14 cases. *Lab. Invest., 42,* 115.

12. Gould, V.E. and Chejfec, G. (1978): Ultrastructural and biochemical analysis of 'undifferentiated' pulmonary carcinomas. *Hum. Path., 9,* 377–384.

13. Hage, E. (1973): Histochemistry and fine structure of bronchial carcinoid tumors. *Virchows Arch. Abt. A. Path. Anat., 361,* 121–128.

14. Hammar, S.P., Bockus, D., Wheelis, R.F. and Hill, L. (1977): Electron microscopic studies of undifferentiated lung tumors. *Chest, 72,* 400.

15. Hattori, S., Matusuda, M., Tateishi, R., Nishihara, M. and Horai, T. (1972): Oat cell carcinoma of the lung: clinical and morphological studies in relation to its histogenesis. *Cancer, 30,* 1014–1024.

16. Hess Jr., F.G., McDowell, E.M., Resau, J.H. and Trump, B.F. (1981): The respiratory epithelium. IX. Validity and reproducibility of revised cytologic criteria of human and hamster respiratory tract tumors. *Acta cytol., 25,* 485.

17. Koss, L.G. (1968): Cancer of the lung. In: *Diagnostic Cytology and its Histopathologic Bases, 2nd ed.* J. B. Lippincott Co., Philadelphia.

18. Kreyberg, L. (1967): Histological typing of lung tumours. *International Histological Classification of Tumours, No. 1.* World Health Organization, Geneva.

19. Lasnitzki, I. (1962): Hypervitaminosis-A in the mouse prostate gland cultured in chemically defined medium. *Exp. Cell Res., 28,* 40–41.

20. Lee, S.H. and Ts'o, T.O. (1963): Histological typing of lung cancers in Hong Kong. *Brit. J. Cancer, 17,* 37–40.

21. Lisa, L.R., Trinidad, S. and Rosenblatt, M.B. (1965): Site of origin, histogenesis and cytostructure of bronchogenic carcinoma. *Amer. J. clin. Path., 44,* 375–384.

22. McDowell, E.M., Barrett, L.A., Glavin, F., Harris, C.C. and Trump, B.F. (1978): The respiratory epithelium. I. Human bronchus. *J. nat. Cancer Inst., 61,* 539–549.

23. McDowell, E.M., Becci, P.J., Schurch, W. and Trump, B.F. (1979): The respiratory epithelium. VII. Epidermoid metaplasia during regeneration of hamster trachea after mechanical injury. *J. nat. Cancer Inst., 62,* 995–1008.

24. McDowell, E.M., McLaughlin, J.S., Merenyi, D.K., Kieffer, R.F., Harris, C.C. and Trump, B.F. (1978): The respiratory epithelium. V. Histogenesis of lung carcinomas in the human. *J. nat. Cancer Inst., 61,* 587–606.

25. McDowell, E.M., Sorokin, S.P., Hoyt, R.F. and Trump, B.F. (1981): An unusual bronchial carcinoid tumor: light and electron microscopy. *Hum. Path., 12,* 338–348.

26. McDowell, E.M. and Trump, B.F. (1981): Pulmonary oat-cell carcinoma showing tripartite differentiation in individual cells. *Hum. Path., 12,* 286–294.

27. McDowell, E.M., Wilson, T.S. and Trump, B.F. (1981): Atypical endocrine tumors of the lung. *Arch. Path. Lab. Med., 105,* 20–28.

28. Pearse, A.G.E. (1966): 5-Hydroxytryptophan uptake by dog thyroid 'C'-cells and its possible significance of polypeptide hormone production. *Nature (Lond.), 116,* 598–600.

29. Prutkin, L. (1975): Mucous metaplasia and gap junctions in the vitamin A acid-treated skin tumor, keratoacanthoma. *Cancer Res., 35,* 364–369.

30. Reznik-Schuller, H. (1976): Proliferation of endocrine (APUD-type) cells during early N-diethylnitrosamine-induced lung carcinogenesis in hamsters. *Cancer Lett., 1,* 255–258.

31. Saladino, A.J., Berezesky, I., Resau, J. and Trump, B.F. (1982): Ionophore A23187 causes hyperplasia in hamster tracheal epithelium. *Fed. Proc.*

32. Schofield, G. (1953): The argentaffin and mucous cells of the human intestine. *Acta anat. (Basel), 18,* 256–272.

33. Shinton, N.K. (1963): The histological classification of lower respiratory tract tumours. *Brit. J. Cancer, 17,* 213–221.

34. Sidhu, G.S. (1979): The endodermal origin of digestive and respiratory tract APUD cells: histopathologic evidence and a review of the literature. *Amer. J. Path., 96,* 5–60.

35. Sorokin, S.P., Hoyt, R.F. and McDowell, E.M. (1981): An unusual bronchial carcinoid tumor analyzed by conjunctive staining. *Hum. Path., 12,* 302–313.

36. Spencer, H. (1968): Carcinoma of the lung. In: *Pathology of the Lung,* pp. 778–869. Pergamon Press, Oxford–New York–Toronto–Sydney–Braunschweig.

37. Steele, V.E. and Nettesheim, P. (1981): Unstable cellular differentiation in adenosquamous cell carcinoma. *J. nat. Cancer Inst., 67,* 149–154.

38. Stoebner, P., Cussac, Y., Porte, A. and Le Gal, Y. (1967): Ultrastructure of anaplastic bronchial carcinomas. *Cancer, 20,* 286–294.

39. Tateishi, J.R. (1973): Distribution of argyrophil cells in adult human lungs. *Arch. Path. Lab. Med., 96,* 198–202.

40. Terzakis, J.A., Sommers, S.C. and Andersson, B. (1972): Neurosecretory appearing cells of human segmental bronchi. *Lab. Invest., 26,* 127–132.

41. Toyashima, K. and Leighton, J. (1975): Vitamin A inhibition of keratinization in rat urinary bladder cancer cell line Nara Bladder Tumors No. 2 in meniscus gradient culture. *Cancer Res., 35,* 1873–1879.

42. Trump, B.F., McDowell, E.M., Becci, P.J., Barrett, L.A., Glavin, F., Kaiser, H.E. and Harris, C.C. (1978): The respiratory epithelium. III. Histogenesis of epidermoid metaplasia and carcinoma in situ in the human. *J. nat. Cancer Inst., 61,* 563–575.

43. Trump, B.F., Berezesky, I.K., Laiho, K.U., Osornio, A.R., Mergner, W.J. and Smith, M.W. (1980): The role of calcium in cell injury: a review. *SEM, 3,* 437–462.

44. Vincent, R.G., Pickren, J.W. and Lane, W.W. (1977): The changing histopathology of lung cancer: a review of 1682 cases. *Cancer, 39,* 1647–1655.

45. Walter, J.B. and Pryce, D.M. (1955): The histology of lung cancer. *Thorax, 10,* 107–116.
46. Warner, T.F.C.S. and Seo, I.S. (1979): Goblet cell carcinoid of the appendix: ultrastructural features and histogenetic aspects. *Cancer, 44,* 1700–1706.
47. Watson, W.L. and Berg, J.W. (1962): Oat cell lung cancer. *Cancer, 15,* 759–768.
48. Willis, R.A. (1961): The incidence and histological types of pulmonary carcinoma, with comments on some fallacies and uncertainties. *Med. J. Aust., 48,* 433–440.
49. Wilson, T.S., McDowell, E.M., McIntire, K.R. and Trump, B.F. (1982): Elaboration of human chorionic gonadotropin by lung tumors: an immunocytochemical study. *Arch. Path. Lab. Med.,* in press.
50. Wolbach, S. and Howe, P. (1925): Tissue changes following deprivation of fat soluble A vitamin. *J. exp. Med., 42,* 753–769.
51. Wong, Y.C. (1975): Mucous metaplasia of the hamster cheek pouch epithelium under hypervitaminosis A. *Exp. mol. Path., 23,* 132–143.
52. Yuspa, S.H., Hawley-Nelson, P., Koehler, B. and Stanley, J.R. (1980): A survey of transformation markers in differentiating epidermal cell lines in culture. *Cancer Res., 40,* 4694–4703.